CLINICAL EPIDEMIOLOGY

the essentials

second edition

CLINICAL EPIDEMIOLOGY

the essentials

second edition

Robert H. Fletcher, M.D., M.Sc.
Professor of Medicine and Epidemiology
The University of North Carolina
Chapel Hill, North Carolina

Suzanne W. Fletcher, M.D., M.Sc.
Professor of Medicine and Epidemiology
The University of North Carolina
Chapel Hill, North Carolina

Edward H. Wagner, M.D., M.P.H.
Director, Center for Health Studies
Group Health Cooperative of Puget Sound
Professor of Health Services
University of Washington
Seattle, Washington

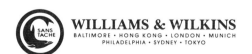
WILLIAMS & WILKINS
BALTIMORE • HONG KONG • LONDON • MUNICH
PHILADELPHIA • SYDNEY • TOKYO

Senior Editor: Nancy Collins
Associate Editor: Carol Eckhart
Copy Editor: Gail Naron Chalew
Text Design: Alice Sellers/Johnson
Illustration Planning: Wayne Hubbel
Production: Raymond E. Reter
Cover Design: Alice Sellers/Johnson

Accurate indications, adverse reactions, and dosage schedules for drugs are provided in this book, but it is possible that they may change. The reader is urged to review the package information data of the manufacturers of the medications mentioned.

Printed in the United States of America

First Edition, 1982

Library of Congress Cataloging in Publication Data

Main entry under title:

Fletcher, Robert H.
  Clinical epidemiology.

  Includes bibliographies and index.
  1. Clinical epidemiology. I. Fletcher, Suzanne W.
II. Wagner, Edward H. (Edward Harris), 1940–
III. Title. [DNLM: 1. Epidemiologic Methods.
WA 950 F614c]
RA652.2.C55F57   1988   616   87-10445
ISBN 0-683-03251-8

12 11   92 93 94

PREFACE TO SECOND EDITION

Five years is not a long time in the 1980s—at least, not for clinical epidemiology. The discipline has undergone an extraordinary growth, both in content and popularity, since the first edition of our book was published in 1982.

In North America, three other books bearing the title "Clinical Epidemiology" have been published over the past few years. Each expresses a somewhat different aspect of the discipline and appeals to somewhat different readers. Journals are presenting more articles that are either about the methods of clinical epidemiology or overtly based on them. Clinicians understand more often the relevance of this point of view about their work, although the extent of understanding varies greatly from place to place. Thus, in North America clinical epidemiology is taking its rightful place as a basic science of clinical medicine.

Clinical epidemiology has also taken hold in other parts of the world. The first edition of our book apparently played some small role in this. Another factor has been the International Clinical Epidemiology Network (INCLEN), a training program of the Rockefeller Foundation that has set hundreds of clinical epidemiologists, including the authors, moving back and forth across the globe to exchange information about doing and teaching clinical epidemiology. Where it has been offered, clinical epidemiology has been well received in developing countries. Clinicians have realized that their practices are no more rational, and their resources for health services certainly no less limited, than ours in North America.

With the growth of clinical epidemiology has come redefinition and expansion of its meaning. Sackett and colleagues refer to it as a "basic science for clinical medicine." Feinstein says that "clinical epidemiology is concerned with studying groups of people to achieve the background evidence needed for clinical decisions in patient care." Weiss calls it the "study of the natural history of disease," and Spitzer defines clinical epidemiology as "the study of determinants and effects of clinical decisions." Others would expand the scope of clinical epidemiology to include clinical decision making, community medicine, clinical economics, health services research, and other related disciplines. There is room for disagreement. What all of these definitions of clinical epidemiology have in common is a respect for the best possible evidence about the actual effectiveness and efficiency of medical care and health services at a time of increasing complexity of what we might do for patients and an increasing recognition that we should not do many things and cannot do all.

In the second edition, we have tried not to make radical changes. After all, the first edition seemed to serve readers well and successive readers are likely to have similar needs, even if the original readers are now more advanced. We have mainly updated examples, redesigned figures, and rewritten a few sections. There are two new chapters. Prevention now stands alone; it is a major issue for clinicians and patients. The final chapter, Summing Up, now concerns the ways in which published research, which often comes to conflicting conclusions, can be weighed and resolved using the methods of a new discipline called meta-analysis. We have tried to accomplish these changes while maintaining the overall size and character of the first edition.

As before, the second time through with this project has given us satisfaction far out of proportion to the effort involved.

R.H.F.
S.W.F.
E.H.W.

PREFACE TO FIRST EDITION

"Clinical epidemiology" is a term none of us had heard during our training. But our need for it became apparent when we first took responsibility for patients. During our "basic science" years in medical school the facts in medicine had seemed formidably embodied in physiologic laws, histologic descriptions, and biochemical pathways. When we became involved in the care of patients, however, we found that the clinical world often operated by a very different set of rules. It was more difficult to determine what was true and not true about clinical medicine, and the ways in which that was judged. At the same time knowing the facts, which until then had been a matter of pure intellectual curiosity, became an urgent necessity. Like other conscientious physicians, we wanted to be reasonably certain that we were doing more good than harm by our actions.

Where could the best possible answers to clinical questions be found?

One approach was to apply the basic principles of human biology. Using knowledge of the chemistry, physiology, and anatomy of disease to solve clinical problems was certainly stimulating and often elegant as well. Sometimes it seemed to be just the right way to proceed. But there were many situations in which this approach fell wide of the mark because of substantial conceptual gaps between the structured experience of basic science and the more complex, open-ended problems arising in the care of patients.

Sometimes we were comfortable taking the word of a trusted authority. But the limitations of this approach were apparent. For one thing, experts often disagreed and so could not all be right. Not only did they disagree about the wisdom of a given diagnostic or therapeutic approach, but also about the validity of the evidence upon which their recommendations were based. Also, most faculty were involved in laboratory research and found it difficult to apply the kind of scientific approaches used in the laboratory to the solution of clinical problems. Evidence that could not be reduced to "hard science" was sometimes viewed by them with uncertainty and suspicion. Moreover, it became clear that experts' personalities and self-interest colored their interpretation of clinical data, as they do for all of us.

So we, like many others, felt compelled to make up our own minds about important clinical questions, referring to published research. It was soon apparent that we had received no formal schooling in this subject. We found ourselves floundering through the medical literature, trying to use intuition, common sense, and good judgment. Although it was clear that we had much to learn, it was not clear what we needed to learn, or how to go about it.

For years, epidemiologists had been asking similar questions about disease, and trying to find the best possible ways to answer them. Epidemiologists paid particular attention to how the validity of human research was affected when it was not possible to perform highly structured experiments, as one might in a laboratory. They had this in common with clinical researchers, and so many of the solutions they devised were highly relevant to clinical medicine. But because epidemiologists and clinicians did not have a history of working together, the flow of information between them had been retarded.

We were fortunate to receive formal training in epidemiology as clinicians, and to be exposed to thoughtful physicians who recognized the potential contribution of that discipline to clinical medicine (see Acknowledgments). With them, we began to develop ways to teach clinicians the application of epidemiologic methods and perspectives to the solution of clinical problems.

When we began to teach our clinical epidemiology course to students and housestaff, we found efforts hindered by the absence of a suitable text. Although a rich array of writings about clinical epidemiology was available, they had not been drawn together, summarized, and simplified in a single book. So we set out to fill this need.

In our book, we have attempted to present the material as simply as possible, and to draw particular attention to major landmarks in a rather cluttered landscape. We recognize that there may be sections in which we have omitted more details than those with a special interest in this field might prefer. We did so for the sake of clarity on the basic issues.

We intend this book for all those who are involved in clinical medicine and want to examine empirical data on their own, in order to make an independent judgment as to the utility of those data in the care of patients. Potential readers include medical students, housestaff, "fully trained" physicians, nurse practitioners, or others engaged in providing care to patients. Because the authors are internists, many of the clinical examples concern medical problems of adults. However, we do not believe that the audience is limited by clinical specialty or seniority. It is our experience, backed by some published studies, that understanding the principles of clinical epidemiology is not concentrated in one or another specialty, and does not necessarily grow with training and experience—as might, for example, knowledge of the content of the medical literature.

Clinical epidemiology contributes to understanding both observations made by individual clinicians and reports of research done by others. Many clinicians do not anticipate a career in research, and so might wonder if learning about research is worthwhile. It seems to us that researchers who collect clinical data and clinicians who use it have a great deal in common. Both have a critical stake in the accuracy of the information. Researchers may need to know more about the particulars of gathering and analyzing the data, and spend more time at it. But clinicians must understand the basic principles of research in order to interpret what is found.

For these reasons, we believe clinical epidemiology is a basic science for clinicians. We rely on it when patient care begins, the evidence is reviewed, and decisions must be made.

ACKNOWLEDGMENTS

In the 5 years since the first edition was published our debt to others has continued to grow.

Bob and Suzanne Fletcher have remained at The University of North Carolina at Chapel Hill. An increasing number of colleagues—students, housestaff, fellows, and faculty—recognize the importance of clinical epidemiology and stimulate us in our daily work. Fellows in the Robert Wood Johnson Foundation's Clinical Scholars Program still play a central role in this process. They have been joined by fellows in the International Clinical Epidemiology Network, a program of the Rockefeller Foundation that includes 31 academic medical centers in 19 developing countries. Strong encouragement from our Schools of Medicine and Public Health has assured that clinical epidemiology is not attached to either clinical or epidemiology departments alone.

Ed Wagner has moved to Seattle, where he directs the Center for Health Studies at Group Health Cooperative of Puget Sound and maintains academic ties in the School of Public Health and Community Medicine, University of Washington. Involvement in a large, managed health care system has reaffirmed the essential role that clinical epidemiologic thinking plays in the rational management of clinical care.

Writing, besides being a deeply satisfying way of communicating with colleagues, is also hard work. Word processors have helped. But we still depended heavily on the help of our staff. We are particularly grateful to Bonnie Parke for her technical assistance, protection of time, and belief in the project itself. Williams & Wilkins has, as before, been both competent and gracious in their support.

Most of all, we appreciate the many people who have offered helpful suggestions, or just plain encouragement, as we have tried to update this book in the face of extraordinary growth of the discipline, without changing its essential character.

CONTENTS

chapter 1

INTRODUCTION

A 51-year-old man sees a physician because of chest pain. He had been well until 2 weeks ago, when he noticed tightness in the center of his chest when he was walking uphill. The tightness stopped after 2 to 3 minutes of rest. A similar discomfort occurred several times since then, sometimes during exercise and sometimes at rest. He smokes one pack of cigarettes per day and has been told in the past that his blood pressure is "a little high." He is otherwise well and takes no medications. However, he is worried about his health, particularly about coronary disease. A complete physical examination and resting electrocardiogram are normal except for a blood pressure of 150/96.

This patient is likely to have many questions. Am I sick? How sure are you? What is causing my illness? How will it affect me? What can be done about it?

The clinician caring for this patient must respond to these questions, considering them in their full complexity. Is the probability of serious, treatable disease high enough to proceed immediately beyond simple explanation and reassurance? How well might various diagnostic tests distinguish among the possible causes of chest pain: angina pectoris, esophageal spasm, muscle strain, anxiety, and the like? Specifically, how helpful will an exercise electrocardiogram be in either confirming or ruling out coronary artery disease? If coronary disease is found, how long can the patient expect to have the pain, and to live? How likely is it that other complications—congestive heart failure, myocardial infarction, or athero-sclerotic disease of other organs—will occur? Will reduction of his risk factors for coronary disease—cigarette smoking and hypertension—reduce his risk? If medications control the pain, should the patient have coronary artery bypass surgery anyway to prevent untimely death?

As clinicians, we use various sources of information to answer these questions: our own experiences, the experiences of our colleagues, and the medical literature. In general, we depend on past observations on other patients to predict what will happen to the patient at hand. The manner in which such observations are made and interpreted frequently determines whether the conclusions we reach are valid.

CLINICAL EPIDEMIOLOGY

Clinical epidemiology is one approach to making and interpreting scientific observations in medicine. *Clinical epidemiology* is the application of epidemiologic principles and methods to problems encountered in clinical medicine. It is a science concerned with counting clinical events occurring in intact human beings, and it uses epidemiologic methods to carry out and analyze the count.

Types of questions addressed by clinical epidemiology are listed in Table 1.1. By and large, these are the same questions confronting the doctor and patient in the example presented at the beginning of this chapter. They are at issue in most doctor-patient encounters.

The clinical events of primary interest in clinical epidemiology are the health outcomes of particular concern to patients and those caring for them (Table 1.2). They are the events doctors try to understand, predict, interpret, and change when caring for patients. Thus, an important dis-

Table 1.1
Clinical Issues and Questions in the Practice of Medicine

ISSUE	QUESTION
Normality/abnormality	Is a person sick or well? What abnormalities are associated with having a disease?
Diagnosis	How accurate are diagnostic tests or strategies used to find a disease?
Frequency	How often does a disease occur?
Risk	What factors are associated with an increased likelihood of disease?
Prognosis	What are the consequences of having a disease?
Treatment	How does treatment change the future course of a disease?
Prevention	Does intervention on people without disease keep disease from arising? Does early detection and treatment improve the course of disease?
Cause	What conditions result in disease? What are the pathogenetic mechanisms of disease?

Table 1.2
Health Outcomes (The Five D's)[a]

Death	A universal health outcome, the timeliness of the event being the issue.
Disease	A combination of symptoms, physical signs, and laboratory test results.
Disability	The functional status of patients in terms of ability to live independently and go about their daily lives at home, work, or recreation.
Discomfort	Uncomfortable symptoms, such as pain, nausea, vertigo, tinnitus, or fatigue.
Dissatisfaction	Emotional and mental states, such as agitation, sadness, or anger.

[a] Some suggest a sixth "D"—destitution—because physicians should be concerned with financial consequences of health care to their patients. Others have pointed out that the five D's emphasize the negative side of health outcomes. Nevertheless, the five D's do remind physicians that clinical events other than death and disease are important.

tinction between clinical epidemiology and other sciences contributing to medicine is that the events of interest in clinical epidemiology can be studied directly only in intact humans and not in animals or parts of humans, such as tissue cultures, pituitary hormones, or red cell membranes.

Many of the methods used to count the clinical events were developed in the field of epidemiology, which has been defined as "the study of the distribution and determinants of disease frequency in man" (1). These methods are the subject of this book.

The basic purpose of clinical epidemiology, then, is to develop and apply methods of clinical observation that will lead to valid clinical conclusions. For clinicians who intend to make up their own minds about the soundness of clinical information, some understanding of this field is as necessary as an understanding of anatomy, pathology, biochemistry, and pharmacology. Indeed, clinical epidemiology is one of the "basic sciences," a foundation on which modern medicine is practiced.

Even so, the principles of clinical epidemiology are not yet second nature to most clinicians. This is partly related to underlying differences between the parent disciplines, clinical medicine and epidemiology. Both are scientific approaches to the causes and consequences of disease in humans. Both have a practical bent, by and large seeking to discover information that can be useful in the control of disease and alleviation of suffering. However, there are some major differences between them as well. When we have explored these differences, we will consider how they can be brought together for the purpose of enriching our understanding of clinical medicine.

Clinical Medicine

As most readers of this book know, clinicians are, by and large, concerned with individual patients. They meet all of their patients personally, take their own histories, and do their own physical examinations. Usually they are not particularly interested in how patients happen to be found in their practices, as opposed to some other medical setting. As a result, clinicians may not feel particularly responsible for other patients, who may be just as sick but have not come to their attention.

Because clinicians bear intense personal responsibility for individual patients, they tend to see what is special about each patient. Thus, it is not surprising that clinicians are often reluctant to lump patients into crude categories of risk, diagnosis, or treatment. Many clinicians are uneasy about uncertainty and reluctant to express it through probabilities. In their work, the stakes commonly are high so that both they and their patients want as much certainty as possible.

Clinical training is largely oriented toward the mechanisms of disease through study of biochemistry, anatomy, physiology, and other basic sciences. These traditional basic sciences are powerful influences in a medical student's formative years, and go on to become the predominant forces in clinical research and publications. This fosters the belief that to understand the detailed processes of disease in individual patients is to understand medicine. The implication is that one can predict the course of disease and select appropriate treatments through knowledge of the mechanisms of disease.

Table 1.3 summarizes both biologic and clinical outcomes for the modern treatment of a patient with acute myocardial infarction. Studies of the biology and pathophysiology of coronary artery disease have greatly increased our understanding of the process. However, for clinical practice such understanding is important only to the extent that these processes are known to be related to the kinds of health outcomes listed in the table.

Epidemiology

Epidemiology is the research discipline concerned with the distribution and determinants of disease in populations. Epidemiologists differ from clinicians in several ways. In contrast to clinicians, epidemiologists are more concerned that their observations represent fairly some defined group of people, or "population." They wish to record the experiences of all members of the group, whether or not they are sick, and whether or not they have come to medical attention. Epidemiologists usually do not personally collect all their data themselves nor do they usually meet the people they study. Because they work with groups rather than with individual patients, epidemiologists are more comfortable with probability.

When epidemiologists study disease, their categories are often crude by clinical standards. They work with such variables as "cigarette smokers" and "nonsmokers" or "sudden death" and "myocardial infarction," even though a myriad of special circumstances is hidden within these classes.

Table 1.3
Biologic and Clinical Outcomes of Medical Care: Treatment of Acute Myocardial Infarction

DISEASE	INTERVENTIONS	OUTCOMES	
		BIOLOGIC	CLINICAL
Acute myocardial infarction	Coronary care Streptokinase Angioplasty	Coronary patency Infarction size Ejection fraction Serum enzymes ECG changes	Death Congestive heart failure Reinfarction Angina
		←————————→ Association known or assumed?	

Epidemiologists are generally more interested in whether something occurs than in how it occurs at a pathogenetic, mechanistic level. They rely in part on an understanding of the mechanism of disease to form hypotheses and then test these hypotheses in human populations. However, if a pathogenetic mechanism is not known, epidemiologists do not necessarily discard a hypothesis. For example, if it can be shown that cigarette smoking in itself is related to cardiovascular disease, and the risk of heart disease decreases when smoking ceases, everything else being equal, the epidemiologist might consider the role of smoking in heart disease largely settled. The more mechanistically inclined biomedical researcher might remain dissatisfied until the causative agent in cigarette smoke is isolated and the pathway by which it causes heart disease is specified.

Because epidemiologists work with groups of individuals, each of which displays unique genetic and environmental characteristics, their stock-in-trade is to know how to deal with variables that are extraneous to the main question at hand. Along the way, they work closely with biostatisticians, who use statistics to summarize the experience of groups, adjust for extraneous differences between groups being compared, and assess whether chance could have determined the findings.

Clinical Epidemiology

Clinical medicine and epidemiology began together. The founders of epidemiology were, for the most part, clinicians. It is only during the past several decades that the two drifted apart, with separate schools, training, journals, and opportunities for employment.

In recent years, clinicians and epidemiologists have become increasingly aware that their fields interrelate and clinical epidemiology began to develop, in recognition of the following:

- In most clinical situations the diagnosis, prognosis and results of treatment are uncertain for individual patients and therefore must be expressed as probabilities.

- Probability for an individual patient is best estimated by referring to past experience with groups of similar patients.
- Because clinical observations are made on people who are free to do as they please, by clinicians with variable skills and prejudices, the observations may be influenced by a variety of systematic errors that can distort the true nature of events and thereby be misleading.
- To deal with these misleading effects, clinical observations should be based on sound scientific principles, including ways to reduce bias and estimate the role of chance.
- These principles are as important to clinicians who wish to be self-sufficient in judging clinical information as they are to researchers who will produce research.

Although the principles of scientific methods are implicit in a great deal of current clinical teaching, they are not a formal part of most medical curricula. But this is changing. A growing understanding of the relevance of epidemiology to clinical medicine is reflected in the recent development of clinical epidemiology courses for medical students, the increased numbers of articles in clinical journals dealing with precepts of clinical epidemiology, and the development of fellowship programs for training clinicians in clinical epidemiology (2).

We hope that this book will contribute to the growth of clinical epidemiology by bringing together, in a few pages, the basic rules of evidence that are important in the clinician's world. We also hope that this book will help clinicians evaluate the constant flow of new medical information. This means that clinicians must learn about the various research designs used in medical research and something about their strengths and pitfalls. With such knowledge, conscientious clinicians can develop skills to help them decide whether new information is worthy of the effort to master it in the first place. For those of us with limited, already oversaturated medical memories, such a skill is indeed useful.

BASIC PRINCIPLES

The basic purpose of clinical epidemiology is to foster methods of clinical observation and interpretation that lead to valid conclusions. This activity is grounded in basic, scientific principles. The remainder of this chapter will introduce these principles. The rest of the book will build on this introduction.

Populations and Samples

In general, *populations* are large groups of people in a defined setting. These include relatively unselected people in the community, the usual population for epidemiologic studies of cause; and groups of people selected because of their attendance in a clinic or hospital or because of a characteristic such as age, race, or the presence of disease. Thus, one speaks of the general population, a hospitalized population, or a population of patients with a specific disease.

A *sample* is a subset of a population and is selected from it. Clinical research is ordinarily carried out on samples. One is interested in the characteristics of the defined population, but must, for practical reasons, describe them through a sample. In doing so, two fundamental questions arise. First, are the conclusions of the research correct for the people in the sample? Second, if so, does the sample represent fairly the population of interest?

Whenever a clinical question is answered by observing people, there are three possible explanations for the answer (Table 1.4). The observation may be incorrect because of bias or chance, or it may be correct.

Bias

Bias is "a process at any stage of inference tending to produce results that depart systematically from the true values" (3).

Suppose, for example, that treatment A is found to work better than treatment B. What kinds of biases might explain the observation? Perhaps A is given to healthier patients than B; then the results could be due to the systematic difference in health between the groups of patients rather than to differences in treatment. Or A might taste better than B so that patients take the drug more regularly. Or A might be a new, very popular drug and B an old one, so that researchers and patients might be more inclined to think that the new drug works better whether or not it really does. All of these are examples of potential biases.

Compared to basic science research, observations on patients (whether for patient care or research) are particularly susceptible to bias. The process tends to be just plain untidy. As participants in a study, human beings have the disconcerting habit of doing as they please and not necessarily what would be required for scientific rigor. When one attempts to conduct

Table 1.4
Possible Explanations for Clinical Observations

BIAS (systematic error)
   Selection bias occurs when comparisons are made between groups of patients that differ with respect to determinants of the outcome other than those under study.
   Measurement bias occurs when the methods of measurement are consistently dissimilar among groups of patients.
   Confounding bias occurs when two factors or processes are associated or "travel together," and the effect of one is confused with or distorted by the effect of the other.
CHANCE (random error)
   Because of random variation, the characteristics of people in a particular sample are different from others in the population from which it was taken.
TRUTH
   The observation is correct. (Accept this explanation only after excluding the others!)

an experiment with them, as one might in a laboratory, things tend to go wrong. Some people refuse to participate, while others drop out or choose another treatment. What is more, some of the most important things about humans—feelings, comfort, performance—are generally more difficult to measure than physical properties, such as blood pressure or serum sodium. The methods of measuring these phenomena are less direct. Then, too, there is the normal inclination of clinicians to believe that their therapies succeed. (Most patients would not want a physician who felt otherwise.) This attitude, so important in the practice of medicine, makes clinical observations particularly vulnerable to bias.

Although dozens of particular biases have been defined, most fall into one of three broad categories (Table 1.4):

1. *Selection bias* **occurs when comparisons are made between groups of patients that differ with respect to determinants of the outcome other than those under study.**

Groups of patients often differ in many ways. If we compare the experience of two groups to decide about the effects of one of their characteristics, free of the others, and the compared groups differ in important ways (other than the factor of interest) at the time of selection, the comparison is biased. As a result little can be concluded about the independent effects of the characteristic of interest.

2. *Measurement bias* **occurs when the methods of measurement are consistently dissimilar among groups of patients.**

An example of a potential measurement bias would be in the use of information taken from medical records to determine if women on birth control pills were more at risk for thromboembolism than those not on "the pill." Suppose a study were made comparing the frequency of oral contraceptive use among women admitted to a hospital because of thrombophlebitis and a group of women admitted for other reasons. It is entirely possible that women, aware of the reported association between estrogens and thrombotic events, might report use of oral contraceptions more completely if they had thrombophlebitis. For the same reasons, clinicians might obtain and record information about oral contraceptive use more thoroughly for women with phlebitis than for those without phlebitis. If so, an observed association between oral contraceptives and thrombophlebitis could be due to the biased way in which the history of exposure was reported.

3. *Confounding bias* **occurs when two factors or processes are associated or "travel together," and the effect of one is confused with or distorted by the effect of the other.**

Example—Is diabetes mellitus, in and of itself, a risk factor for atherosclerotic disease? The clinical manifestations of atherosclerosis—myocardial infarction, sudden death, peripheral vascular disease, stroke, and others—are all more likely to occur in patients with diabetes. But other risk factors for cardiovascular disease—blood pressure, weight, and serum cholesterol—are all higher in diabetics. Perhaps the increased risk in diabetics is because of these other factors, rather than the diabetes itself. However, even after the effects of these other factors are taken into account, diabetics are at increased risk (4).

Example—Several studies have shown that serum triglyceride levels (TG) are associated with risk for coronary heart disease (CHD): the higher the TG, the higher the risk. Because of this, clinicians have screened for TG and attempted to lower TG when it was elevated. This might be helpful if TG were an independent cause of CHD. But other known causes of CHD, particularly elevated serum cholesterol levels and reduced levels of high density lipoprotein, are related to both serum triglycerides and CHD. When the contribution of these other factors is removed, the relationship between TG and CHD no longer is present. It seems unlikely, therefore, that TG is an independent cause of CHD; its relationship to CHD is confounded with other factors that are independent causes (5) (Fig. 1.1).

It should be apparent that selection bias and confounding bias are not mutually exclusive. They are described separately, however, because they present problems at different points in a clinical observation or study. Selection bias is at issue primarily when patients are chosen for observation, and so it is important in the design of a study. Confounding bias comes to the fore in analysis of the data, once the observations have been made.

Often in the same study more than one bias operates, as in the following hypothetical example.

Example—A study was done to determine whether regular exercise lowers the risk of CHD. An exercise program was offered to employees of a plant, and the rate of subsequent coronary events was compared among employees who volunteered for the program and those who did not volunteer. Coronary events were determined by means of regular voluntary checkups, including a careful history and electrocardiogram, and review of routine health records. The group that exercised had lower rates of CHD. However, they also smoked cigarettes less.

In this example, selection bias could be present if volunteers for the exercise program were, for any reason, at lower risk for coronary disease even before the program began—e.g., because they had lower serum lipids or less family history of coronary disease. Measurement bias might have occurred because the exercise group stood a better chance of having a coronary event detected, inasmuch as more of them were likely to be

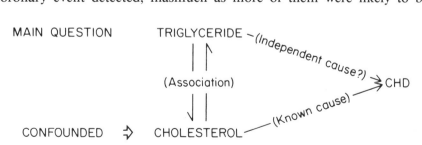

Figure 1.1. Confounding bias. Serum triglyceride is a risk factor for coronary heart disease (CHD) but not independently of serum cholesterol.

examined routinely. Finally, the conclusion that exercise lowered the risk of coronary disease might be the result of a confounding bias if the association between exercise and coronary events in this particular study resulted from the fact that smoking cigarettes is a risk factor for coronary disease and the exercise group smoked less.

A distinction must be made between the potential for bias and the actual presence of bias in a particular study. It is first necessary to recognize the importance of bias and to know where and how to look for it and what can be done about it. But one should not stop there. It is also necessary to determine whether bias is in fact present and how large it is likely to be, in order to decide whether it is important enough to change the conclusions of the study in a clinically meaningful way.

Chance

Observations about disease are ordinarily made on a sample of patients rather than all those with the disease in question. A single set of observations, even if selected in an unbiased way, may misrepresent the truth because of error arising from random variation. In fact, actual observations on a single sample are unlikely to correspond exactly to the true state of affairs in the larger group of all patients. However, if the observations were repeated on many such samples, they would be found to vary about the true value. The divergence of an observation on a sample from the true population value, due to chance alone, is called *random variation.*

We are all familiar with chance as an explanation for why a coin does not come up heads exactly 50% of the time when it is flipped, say, 100 times. The same influence, random variation, applies when assessing the effects of treatments A and B, discussed earlier. Suppose all biases were removed from a study of the relative effects of two treatments. Suppose, further, that the two treatments were, in reality, equally effective, each improving about 50% of the patients treated. Even so, because of chance alone, a single study involving small numbers of patients in each treatment group might easily find A improving a much larger proportion of patients than B, or vice versa.

Chance can affect all of the steps involved in clinical observations. In the assessment of treatments A and B, random variation can occur in the sampling of patients for the study, the selection of treatment groups, and the measurements made on the groups.

Unlike bias, which deflects values in one direction or another, random variation is as likely to result in observations above the true value as below. As a consequence, the mean of many unbiased observations on samples tends to correspond to the true value in the population, even though the results of individual small samples may not.

Statistics can be used to estimate the probability of chance or random variation accounting for clinical results. A knowledge of statistics can also help reduce that probability. It is important, however, to understand that random variation cannot be totally eliminated. Chance should always be considered when assessing the results of clinical observations.

Relationship between Bias and Chance

The relationship between bias and chance is illustrated in Figure 1.2. The measurement of diastolic blood pressure on a single patient is taken as an example. True blood pressure can be obtained by an intra-arterial cannula, and multiple readings are illustrated as all being 80 mm Hg. But this method is not possible for routine measurements. Blood pressure is ordinarily measured indirectly, using a sphygmomanometer. The simpler instrument is prone to error, or deviations from the true value. In the example, this is represented by all of the sphygmomanometer readings falling to the right of the true value. The deviation of sphygmomanometer readings to the right (bias) may have several explanations—e.g., a poorly calibrated sphygmomanometer, a wrong cuff size, or a deaf clinician. Bias could also result if different sounds were chosen to represent diastolic blood pressure. The usual end points—phase IV and phase V Korotkoff sounds—tend to be above and below the true diastolic pressure, respectively; and even that is unpredictable in obese people. Individual blood pressure readings would also be subject to error because of random variation in measurement, as illustrated by the spread of the sphygmomanometer readings around the mean value (90 mm Hg).

The two sources of error—bias and chance—are not mutually exclusive. In most situations, both are present. The main reason for distinguishing between the two is that they are handled differently.

Bias, in theory, can be prevented by conducting clinical investigations

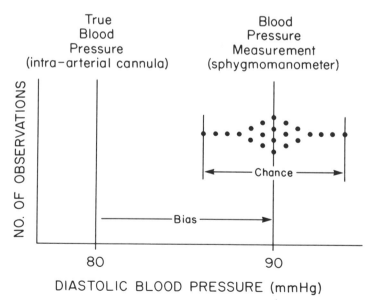

Figure 1.2. Relationship between bias and chance. Blood pressure measurements by intra-arterial cannula and sphygmomanometer.

properly or corrected through proper data analysis. If not eliminated, bias often can be detected by the discerning reader. Most of this book is about how to recognize, avoid, or minimize bias.

Chance cannot be eliminated, but its influence can be reduced by proper design of research, and the remaining error estimated by statistics. Statistics can also help remove the effects of known biases. However, no amount of statistical treatment can correct for unknown biases in data. Some would go so far as to prefer that statistics not be applied to data vulnerable to bias because of poor research design, for fear of giving false respectability to misleading work.

Validity

A clinical observation is valid if it corresponds to the true state of the phenomenon being measured. For the observation to be valid, it must be neither biased nor incorrect due to chance. There are two general kinds of validity—internal validity and external validity, or generalizability.

Internal validity is the degree to which the results of an observation are correct for the patients being studied. It is "internal" because it applies to the particular conditions of the particular group of patients being observed, and not necessarily to others. The internal validity of clinical observations is determined by how well they are carried out, and is threatened by all of the biases and random variation discussed previously. For a clinical observation to be useful, internal validity is a necessary but not sufficient condition.

External validity (*generalizability*) is the degree to which the results of an observation hold true in other settings. For an individual physician, it is an answer to the question: "Assuming that the results of a study are true, do they apply to my patient as well?" Generalizability expresses the validity of assuming that patients in a study are comparable to other patients.

An unimpeachable study, with high internal validity, may be totally misleading when the results are generalized to certain other patients. This is because of yet another bias, sampling bias. *Sampling bias* occurs when observations and conclusions based on a sample of people are generalized to other groups who are not similar.

Example—Sampling bias was demonstrated in studies of febrile seizures in children. Because febrile seizures commonly occur in childhood (reportedly in 2–4% of all children) it is important to know if such seizures recur. If they frequently recur, treatment with anticonvulsant therapy may be worth considering. On the other hand, if febrile seizures are usually one-time phenomena, reassurance of the parents is in order.

Figure 1.3 shows the recurrence rates of seizures among children reported in various studies, according to how the children were chosen for the study. On the left, population-based studies followed up all children who had febrile seizures in the defined population. The recurrence rates reported in these studies were all very low. Clinic-based studies, shown on the right of Figure 1.3, described recurrence

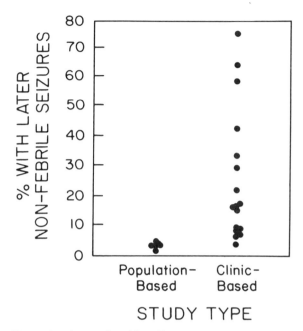

Figure 1.3. Example of sampling bias. Recurrent seizures in infants with febrile seizures in population-based and clinic-based studies. (Redrawn from Ellenberg JH, Nelson KB: Sample selection and the natural history of disease. Studies of febrile seizures. *JAMA* 243:1337–1340, 1980.)

rates in children attending hospital clinics or specialty referral units, and reported much higher recurrence rates.

Applying the results of referral hospital studies to community practices would result in falsely high estimates of the likelihood of recurring seizures. On the other hand, using the conclusion of the population-based studies when discussing the prognosis of febrile seizures with the parents of a child referred to a pediatric neurology unit might also be inaccurate, this time in the opposite direction (6).

The generalizability of clinical observations, even those with internal validity, is a matter of opinion about which reasonable people might disagree. For example, the Veterans Administration (VA) study of hypertension treatment was carried out with special attention to potential biases and chance. As a result, the internal validity of this study, with its conclusion that lowering blood pressure decreased risk of death and severe morbid events in the particular patients in the study, is generally accepted (7). But the study was confined to men. Some clinicians were willing to use the results of this study to guide decisions about treatment of women. Others, more skeptical because of known differences in the frequency of cardiovascular disease between men and women, were unwilling to do so. The VA study itself held no solution to this disagreement. The only way to resolve the dispute was to collect data on women with hypertension. Such studies have subsequently been done and found similar results for women.

Generalizability can rarely be dealt with satisfactorily in any one study. Even a defined, geographically based population is a biased sample of larger populations; for example, hospital patients are biased samples of county residents, counties of states, states of regions, and so on. Adding additional centers may improve generalizability, but not settle the issue.

Usually, the best a researcher can do about generalizability is to ensure internal validity, have the study population fit the research question, and avoid studying groups so unusual that experience with them generalizes to few other settings. It then remains for other studies, in other settings, to extend generalizability.

Because most clinical studies take place in medical centers and because patients in such centers usually overrepresent the serious end of the disease spectrum, sampling bias in clinical research tends to exaggerate the serious nature of disease.

The relationships among internal and external validity, bias, and chance are shown in Figure 1.4.

DESCRIPTION AND COMPARISON

Clinical research can simply describe the frequency of a clinical phenom-

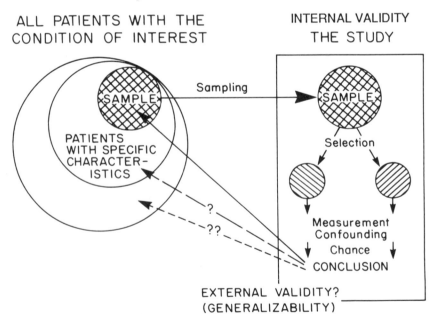

Figure 1.4. Relationships among internal and external validity, bias, and chance.

enon. For example, one might ask: What proportion of young women with dysuria have bacterial cystitis?; or what is the rate of stroke in people with carotid bruits? Simple descriptions are useful in their own right. They guide clinical predictions.

More often, a comparison is also made: Is cystitis more common in women with, as opposed to without, pyuria?; or are strokes more common in people with carotid bruits, compared to people without? In this process, one is looking for an association (or possibly a cause-and-effect relationship) between two or more factors.

When comparisons are made, bias and chance are acknowledged by two modifiers to the basic question: Is X associated with Y (a) everything else being equal? (*bias*); and (b) more often than would have been expected by chance alone? (*chance*)

INFORMATION AND DECISIONS

The primary concern of this book is the quality of information and its correct interpretation. Making decisions is another matter. True, good decisions depend on good information; but they involve a great deal more as well, including value judgments and the weighing of competing risks and benefits.

In recent years, various methods for "quantitative" decision making have become popular. Among these are decision analysis, cost-benefit analysis, and cost-effectiveness analysis. They involve presenting the decision-making process in an explicit way, so that the components of the decision and the consequences of assigning various values to them can be examined. Some aspects of decision analysis, such as evaluation of diagnostic tests, are included in this book. However, we have elected not to go deeply into medical decision making itself. Our justification is that ultimately decisions are only as good as the information used to make them, and we have found enough to say about the essentials of collecting and interpreting clinical information to fill a book. Readers who wish to delve more deeply into decision analysis can begin with some of the readings suggested at the end of this chapter.

ORGANIZATION OF BOOK

In most textbooks of clinical medicine, information about disease is presented as answers to traditional clinical questions, as outlined in Table 1.1. On the other hand, most books about clinical investigation are organized around research strategies: clinical trials, surveys, case-control studies, etc. This way of organizing a book may serve those who would perform clinical research, but it is often awkward for clinicians. As a result, clinicians do not have a comprehensive source of information about the basic structure of clinical observations as it relates to clinical practice, as they do for the clinical relevance of the basic sciences.

This book is written for clinicians who wish to understand the methods of clinical observation and research. We have not written primarily for those who would perform clinical research, but for all the rest who depend on it. However, we believe that the basic needs of those who create and those who use clinical research findings are similar.

We have organized the book primarily according to the clinical questions surrounding doctor-patient encounters. Figure 1.5 illustrates how these questions correspond to the book chapters, taking lung cancer as an example. The questions relate to the entire natural history of disease, from the time nondiseased people are first exposed to risk, through when some acquire the disease and emerge as patients, until the end results of disease are manifest.

In each chapter, strategies used to answer the clinical questions are described. Occasionally, a given strategy, such as a cohort study, may be

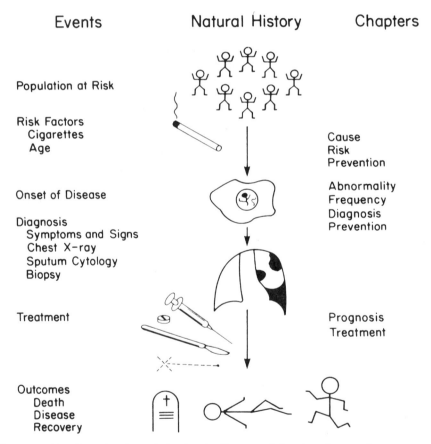

Figure 1.5. Organization of the book, illustrated for the disease lung cancer. Issues covered in the chapters on chance and cause relate to the entire progression of disease.

useful in answering several clinical questions. For the purposes of presentation, we have arbitrarily discussed these strategies primarily in one chapter. But it is important to keep in mind that given clinical epidemiologic methods may be applicable to more than one clinical question. When this is so, we have attempted to refer to these methods in other relevant chapters.

REFERENCES

1. Sackett DL, Haynes RB, Tugwell P: *Clinical Epidemiology. A Basic Science for Clinical Medicine.* Boston, Little, Brown, and Co, 1985.
2. Fletcher RH, Fletcher SW: Clinical epidemiology. A new discipline for an old art. *Ann Intern Med* 99:401–403, 1983.
3. Murphy EA. *The Logic of Medicine.* Baltimore, Johns Hopkins University Press, 1976.
4. Dawber TR: *The Framingham Study. The Epidemiology of Atherosclerotic Disease.* Cambridge, MA, Harvard University Press, 1980.
5. Hulley SB, Rosenman RH, Bawol RD, Brand RJ: Epidemiology as a guide to clinical decisions: The association between triglyceride and coronary heart disease. *N Engl J Med* 302:1383–1389, 1980.
6. Ellenberg JH, Nelson KB: Sample selection and the natural history of disease: Studies of febrile seizures. *JAMA* 243:1337–1340, 1980.
7. Veterans Administration Cooperative Study Group on Antihypertensive Agents. Effects of treatment on morbidity in hypertension. *JAMA* 202:1028–1034, 1967 and 213:1143–1152, 1970.

SUGGESTED READINGS

Cebul RD, Beck LH (eds): *Teaching Clinical Decision Making.* New York, Praeger, 1985.
Chalmers AF: *What is This Thing Called Science? An Assessment of the Nature and Status of Science and Its Methods,* ed 2. Queensland, Queensland University Press, 1982.
Department of Clinical Epidemiology and Biostatistics, McMaster University Health Sciences Centre. Clinical Epidemiology Rounds: How to read clinical journals I–V. *Can Med Assoc J* 124:555–558, 703–710, 869–872, 985–990, 1156–1162, 1981.
Feinstein AR: *Clinical Judgment.* Baltimore, Williams & Wilkins, 1967.
Feinstein AR: Why clinical epidemiology *Clin Res* 20:821–825, 1972.
Feinstein AR: *Clinical Biostatistics.* St. Louis, CV Mosby, 1977.
Feinstein AR: *Clinical Epidemiology. The Architecture of Clinical Research.* Boston, Little, Brown, and Co, 1985.
Fletcher RH, Fletcher SW: Clinical epidemiology. A new discipline for an old art. *Ann Intern Med* 99:401–403, 1983.
Hulley SB, Cummings SR: *Designing Clinical Research. An Epidemiologic Approach.* Baltimore: Williams & Wilkins, in press.
Jenicek M, Cléroux R: *Épidémiologie Clinique. Clinimétrie.* St-Hyacinthe, Quebec, Edisem, 1985.
Michael M III, Boyce WT, Wilcox AJ: *Biomedical Bestiary: An Epidemiologic Guide to Flaws and Fallacies in the Medical Literature.* Boston: Little, Brown and Co, 1984.
Research Development Committee, Society for Research and Education in Primary Care Internal Medicine: Clinical research methods: An annotated bibliography. *Ann Intern Med* 99:419–424, 1983.
Riegelman RK: *Studying a Study and Testing a Test. How to Read the Medical Literature.* Boston, Little, Brown and Co, 1981.
Sackett DL: Clinical epidemiology. *Am J Epidemiol* 89:125–128, 1969.
Sackett DL: Bias in analytic research. *J Chron Dis* 32:51–63, 1979.
Sackett DL: Three cheers for clinical epidemiology. *Int J Epidemiol* 13:117–119, 1984.

Sackett DL, Haynes RB, Tugwell P: *Clinical Epidemiology. A Basic Science for Clinical Medicine.* Boston, Little, Brown, and Co, 1985.

Sox HC Jr, Blatt M, Higgins MC, Marton KI: *Medical Decision Making.* London, Butterworths, in press.

Spitzer WO. Clinical epidemiology. *J Chron Dis* 39:411–415, 1986.

Weinstein MC, Fineberg HV, Elstein AS, Frazier HS, Neuhauser D, Neutra RR, McNeil BJ: *Clinical Decision Analysis.* Philadelphia, WB Saunders, 1980.

Weiss NS. *Clinical Epidemiology: The Study of the Outcome of Illness.* New York, Oxford University Press, 1986.

APPENDIX 1.1. QUESTIONS THAT APPLY TO MOST CLINICAL RESEARCH

1. The research question
   a. What general *kind of clinical question* is the research intended to answer: abnormality, diagnosis, frequency, risk, prognosis, treatment, or prevention? (Appropriate research design depends on the question.)
   b. What is the *specific question?*
2. Generalizability/importance
   a. Were the *patients* in the study like the ones I see?
   b. If *predictive factors* (risk or prognostic factors, prevention, or therapeutic interventions) were studied, are they present in my setting?
   c. Were the *outcomes* important to my patients and me?
3. Bias
   a. Could the observed findings be the result of bias? (See appendices at the end of Chapters 3, 4, 6, and 10.)
   b. If bias is present, is it large enough to affect the conclusions?
4. Chance
   a. If the study found a difference, how likely is it to have occurred by chance alone (alpha error), either for single comparison (probability of error estimated by a *p* value) or as a result of multiple comparisons?
   b. If the study found no difference, how likely was it to detect a clinically important difference? (*statistical power*)
   c. If the study reports a rate, or difference in rates, what is the *precision* of the observation—the range that is likely to include the true rate (confidence intervals).

chapter 2

ABNORMALITY

Clinicians spend a great deal of time distinguishing "normal" from "abnormal" biology. When confronted with something grossly different from the usual, there is of course little difficulty telling the two apart. We are all familiar with pictures in classic textbooks of physical diagnosis showing obvious examples of massive hepatosplenomegaly, goiter, or elephantiasis. We can take no particular pride in recognizing this degree of abnormality. More often, however, clinicians must make subtler distinctions between normal and abnormal. Is fleeting chest pain pleurisy or inconsequential? Is a soft systolic heart sound a sign of valvular heart disease or an innocent murmur? Is a slightly elevated serum alkaline phosphatase evidence for liver disease, asymptomatic Paget's disease, or nothing at all?

Decisions about what is abnormal are most difficult among unselected patients usually found outside the hospital. When patients have already been screened and selected for special attention, as is the case in most referral centers, it is usually clear that something is wrong. The task is then to refine a description of the problem and treat it. In primary care settings, however, subtle manifestations of disease are freely mixed with more everyday complaints of healthy people, and it is not possible to pursue all of those complaints aggressively. Which of many patients with abdominal pain have self-limited gastroenteritis and which have early appendicitis? Which patients with sore throat and hoarseness have a "garden variety" pharyngitis and which the rare but potentially lethal *Haemophilus* epiglottitis? These are examples of how difficult, and important, distinguishing various kinds of abnormality can be.

The point of distinguishing normal from abnormal is to separate out those observations that should be considered for action from those that can be discounted. Observations considered normal are usually described as "within normal limits," "unremarkable," or "noncontributory" and remain buried in the body of a medical history. The abnormal findings are set out under a problem list, "impressions," or "diagnoses" and are the basis for action.

Simply calling clinical findings normal or abnormal is undoubtedly crude and results in some misclassification. The justification for taking this approach is that there are times when it is impractical, or unnecessary, to consider the raw data in all their detail. As Bertrand Russell put it, "To be perfectly intelligible one must be inaccurate, and to be perfectly accurate, one must be unintelligible." Physicians usually choose to err on the side of being intelligible—to themselves and others—even at the expense of some accuracy. Another reason for simplifying data is that each aspect of a physician's work ends in a decision; to pursue evaluation or to wait; to select a treatment or reassure. Under these circumstances some sort of classification becomes necessary.

Table 2.1 is an example of how relatively simple expressions of abnormality are derived from more complex clinical data. On the left is a typical problem list, a statement of the patient's important medical problems. On the right are some of the data upon which the decisions to call them problems are based. Conclusions from the data, represented by the problem list, are by no means noncontroversial. The mean of the four diastolic blood pressure measurements is 94 mm Hg. Some might argue that this level of blood pressure does not justify the label "hypertension," because it is not particularly high and there are some disadvantages to telling patients they are sick and giving them pills. Others might consider the label fair, considering that this level of blood pressure is associated with an increased risk of cardiovascular disease, and that the risk may be reduced by treatment. Although crude, the list serves as a basis for decisions— about diagnosis, prognosis, treatment—and decisions must be made, whether actively or passively.

This chapter will present some of the ways clinicians distinguish normal from abnormal. In order to do so, first it will be necessary to consider how biologic phenomena are measured, described, and distributed among un-

Table 2.1

Summarization of Clinical Data: A Patient's Problem List and the Data on Which It is Based

PROBLEM LIST	RAW DATA			
1. Hypertension	Several blood pressure readings: 170/102, 150/86, 166/92, 172/96			
2. Diabetes mellitus	Glucose tolerance test			
	Time (hours)	0	½	1	2
	Plasma glucose	110	190	170	140
	(mg/100 ml)			
3. Renal insufficiency	Serum chemistries: Creatinine 2.7 mg/100 ml Urea nitrogen 40 mg/100 ml Bicarbonate 18 mEq/liter			

selected people. Then it will be possible to consider how these data are used as a basis for value judgments about what is worth calling abnormal.

CLINICAL MEASUREMENT

There are three principal scales (ways of expressing measurements) used for measuring clinical phenomena: nominal, ordinal, and interval.

Data that can only be placed into categories, without any inherent order, are called *nominal*. Relatively few clinical phenomena can be categorized with such sharp distinction that they might be considered truly normal. Most are determined by a small set of genes (e.g., tissue antigens, sex, inborn errors of metabolism) or are dramatic, discrete events (e.g., death, dialysis, or surgery). Data like these can be placed in categories without much concern about misclassification. It only remains to determine the clinical significance of belonging to one of the categories. Data that can be divided into two unordered categories (present/absent, yes/no, alive/dead) are called *dichotomous.*

Clinical data that possess some inherent ordering or rank—small to large, good to bad, etc—but for which the size of the intervals cannot be specified, are called *ordinal* data. Some clinical examples include: mild-moderate-severe dyspnea, 1+ to 4+ leg edema, and grades $\frac{I}{VI}$ to $\frac{VI}{VI}$ murmurs.

For *interval* scales, there is an inherent order, and the difference between successive values is always the same (1). Interval data have also been called *numerical* (2) or *dimensional* (3). There are two general types of interval scales. *Continuous* scales can take on any value in a continuum. Examples include most serum chemistries, weight, blood pressure, and partial pressure of oxygen in arterial blood. *Discrete* scales can take on only specific values and are expressed as counts. Example of discrete data are heart rate, number of seizures per month, and number of white blood cells in urine per microscopic high-power field.

Reports of continuous variables may in practice be confined to a limited number of points on the continuum, often integers, because that is an honest representation of the precision of the measurement. For example, the blood glucose may in fact be 193.2846573. . . mg/100 ml but simply reported as 193 mg/100 ml. But this does not change the fact that the data can fall anywhere on the continuum.

It is for ordinal and interval data that the question arises: Where does normal leave off and abnormal begin? When, for example, does a large normal prostate become too large to be considered normal? We are free to choose any cutoff point. Some of the reasons for the choices will be considered later in this chapter.

"HARD" AND "SOFT" MEASUREMENTS

Although evaluation of symptoms plays a major role in clinical medicine, ways of measuring symptoms have received relatively little attention in the medical literature.

Because of their selection and training, physicians value the kind of precise measurements the physical and biologic sciences afford. Sometimes, however, this approach is at the expense of clinical relevance, and has distorted the "picture" of medicine presented by published research.

As Feinstein puts it (4):

The term "hard" is usually applied to data that are reliable and preferably dimensional (e.g., laboratory data, demographic data, and financial costs). But clinical performance, convenience, anticipation, and familial data are "soft." They depend on subjective statements, usually expressed in words rather than numbers, by the people who are the observers and the observed.

To avoid such soft data, the results of treatment are commonly restricted to laboratory information that can be objective, dimensional, and reliable—but it is also dehumanized. If we are told that the serum cholesterol is 230 mg per 100 ml, that the chest X-ray shows cardiac enlargement, and that the electrocardiogram has Q waves, we would not know whether the treated object was a dog or a person. If we were told that capacity at work was restored, that the medicine tasted good and was easy to take, and that the family was happy about the results, we would recognize a human set of responses.

With suitable attention given to the scientific challenges, the quality of soft data could be hardened.

VALIDITY AND RELIABILITY

Two concepts are used to describe the quality of measurements, regardless of the scale on which they are expressed. These concepts are called validity and reliability.

Validity

As pointed out in Chapter 1, *validity* is the degree to which the results of a measurement correspond to the true state of the phenomenon being measured. Another word for validity is *accuracy.*

For clinical observations that can be measured by physical means, it is relatively easy to establish validity. The observed measurement is compared to some accepted standard. For example, serum sodium can be measured on an instrument recently calibrated against solutions made up with known concentrations of sodium. Similarly, the validity of a physical finding can be established by the results of surgery or an autopsy.

For other clinical measurements, however, no physical standards of validity exist. Among these are pain, nausea, dyspnea, anxiety, and fear.

In clinical medicine, information about these phenomena is obtained as part of an interview. A more formal and standardized approach, used in clinical research, is a questionnaire. Groups of questions are designed to measure specific phenomena (feelings, attitudes, knowledge, beliefs) called "constructs." Responses to all questions concerning a construct are converted to numbers and grouped together to form a "scale."

There are three general strategies for establishing the validity of measurements that cannot be confirmed directly using the physical senses. *Content validity* is the extent to which a particular method of measurement includes all of the dimensions of the construct being measured, and nothing more. For example, a scale for measuring pain would have construct validity if it included questions about aching, throbbing, burning, and stinging, but not about pressure, itching, nausea, tingling, and the like.

Construct validity is affirmed if the results from a scale vary according to the presence of other established indicators of pain—for example, sweating, moaning, asking for pain medications—that are known to be associated with pain. Alternatively, one might see if responses on the scale bear a predictable relation to pain of known severity: mild pain from minor abrasion, moderate pain from ordinary headache and peptic ulcer, and severe pain from renal colic.

Criterion validity is established by showing that the measurement predicts a directly observable phenomenon. For example, an observation that chest pain is the result of an acute myocardial infarction is confirmed if a documented infarction follows directly on it.

With these and other indirect strategies, one can attempt to build a case for or against the validity of a scale, under the conditions in which it is used. Thus, validity is not, as is often asserted, either present or absent; one can only believe that a scale is more or less valid as a result of these strategies. Although the process of validating a scale may not be as reassuring as confirming the accuracy of a laboratory test, it is better to try than simply to assume that a question measures what we hope it does.

Reliability

Reliability is the extent to which repeated measurements of a relatively stable phenomenon fall closely to each other. *Reproducibility* and *precision* are other words for this property.

The relationships between reliability and validity are shown in Figure 2.1. It is possible to have an instrument (e.g., laboratory instrument or questionnaire) that is on the average valid (accurate) but not reliable, because its results are widely scattered about the true value. On the other hand, an instrument can be very reliable, but systematically off the mark (inaccurate).

VARIATION

Clinical measurements can take on a range of values, depending on the circumstances in which they are made. Sometimes this variation can be so great that any given observation or small set of observations is likely to present a misleading representation of what it is being measured. To avoid erroneous conclusions from data, clinicians should be be aware of the

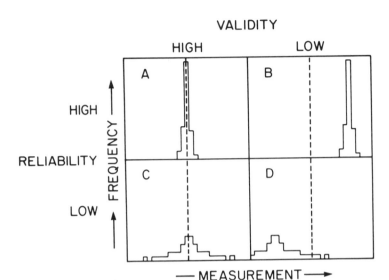

Figure 2.1. Validity and reliability *A*, High validity and reliability. *B*, Low validity and high reliability. *C*, High validity and low reliability. *D*, Low validity and reliability. The *dotted lines* represent the true values.

reasons for variation in a given situation, and which are likely to play a large part, a small part, or no part at all in what has been observed.

Sources of Variation

How does variation arise? The conditions that contribute to overall variation include the act of measurement, the biologic differences within individuals from time to time, and the biologic differences from person to person (Table 2.2). The variation from these sources is cumulative, so that observations subject to any one source are also subject to the others that precede it. This way of thinking about variation gives us a means of sorting out which sources are likely to apply in a given situation, how much they have contributed to the observed data, and how they might be reduced.

Measurement Variation

All observations are subject to variation resulting from measurement because of the performance of the instruments and observers involved in making the measurement. It is possible to reduce this source of variation by making measurements with great care and following standard protocols. However, when measurements involve human judgment, rather than machines, variation can be particularly large and difficult to control.

Example—Fetal heart rate is often monitored by auscultation, which is subject to observer error. Electronic monitoring gives the true rate. Fetal heart rates that

Table 2.2
Sources of Variation

SOURCE	DEFINITION	
Measurement		
Instrument	The means of making the measurement	
Observer	The person making the measurement	
Biologic		Cumulative
Within individuals	Changes in people with time and situation	
Among individuals	Biologic differences from person to person	

are unusually high or low are markers of fetal distress, possibly calling for early delivery.

Day et al. compared fetal heart rates obtained by hospital staff, by auscultation, to rates by electronic monitoring (Fig. 2.2) (5). When the true fetal heart rate was in the normal range, rates by auscultation were evenly distributed about the true value—that is, there was random error only. But when the true fetal heart rate was unusually high or low, rates by auscultation were biased toward normal. Low rates tended to be reported as higher than the true rates, and high rates as lower than the true rates.

This study illustrates both random and systematic errors in clinical observations. In this case, the bias toward normal rates might have arisen because hospital staff hoped the fetus was well and were reluctant to undertake a major intervention based on their observations.

Variations in measurements also arise because measurements are made on only a sample of the phenomenon being described. Often the *sampling fraction*—the fraction of the whole that is included in the sample—is very small. A liver biopsy represents only about 1/100,000 of the liver. Because so little of the whole is examined, there is room for considerable variation from one sample to another. If measurements are made by several different methods (e.g., different laboratories, different technicians, or different instruments) some of the determinations may be unreliable and manifest systematic differences from the correct value, contributing to the spread of values obtained.

Biologic Variation

Variation also arises because of biologic changes within individuals over time. Most biologic phenomena change from moment to moment. A measurement at a point in time is a sample of measurements during a period of time and may not represent the "true" value of these measurements.

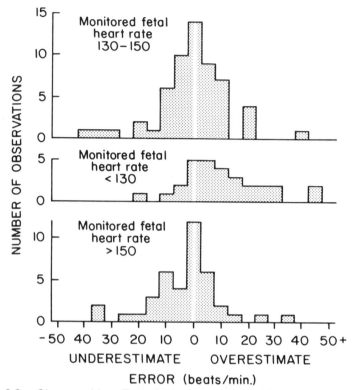

Figure 2.2. Observer bias. Error in reporting of fetal heart rate according to whether the true rate, determined by electronic monitor, is within the normal range, low, or high. (Redrawn from Day E, Maddern L, Wood C: Auscultation of foetal heart rate: an assessment of its error and significance. *Br Med J* 4:422–424, 1968.)

Example—Clinicians usually estimate the frequency of ventricular premature depolarization (VPD) to help determine the need for and effectiveness of treatment by making relatively brief observations—perhaps feeling a pulse for 1 minute or reviewing an electrocardiogram (as little as 10 seconds of observation). However, the frequency of VPDs in a given patient varies with time. To obtain a larger sample of VPD rate, a portable (Holter) monitor is sometimes used. But monitoring even for extended periods of time can be misleading. Figure 2.3 shows observations on one patient with VPDs, similar to others studied. VPDs per hour varied from less than 20 to 380, according to day and time of day. The authors concluded: "To distinguish a reduction in VPD frequency attributable to therapeutic intervention rather than biologic or spontaneous variation alone required a greater than 83% reduction in VPD frequency if only two 24-hour monitoring periods were compared . . ." (6).

Finally, variation arises because of differences among subjects. Biologic differences among people predominate in many situations. For example,

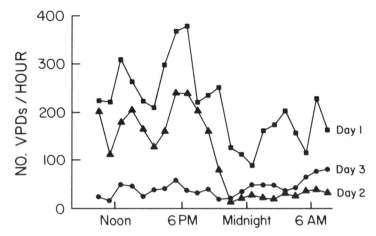

Figure 2.3.   Biologic variability. The number of ventricular premature depolarizations (VPDs) for one untreated patient on 3 consecutive days. (Redrawn from Morganroth J, Michelson EL, Horowitz LN, Josephson ME, Pearlman AS, Dunkman WB: Limitations of routine long-term electrocardiographic monitoring to assess ventricular ectopic frequency. *Circulation* 58:408–414, 1978.)

several studies have shown that a casual blood pressure, although subject to all other forms of variation, is highly predictive of subsequent cardiovascular disease.

Sometimes important sources of variation may be ignored because it is inconvenient, even threatening, to acknowledge them. For example, when caring for an ambulatory patient with ventricular arrhythmia, it would be preferable to use simple clinical observations, such as feeling the pulse, to guide clinical decisions. Protracted monitoring is just not feasible on a day-to-day basis. Also, clinicians want one or another of their treatments to work, and this perfectly normal feeling may influence how they interpret the different rates they observe. As a result, the enormous variation in VPD rate within subjects may be too readily discounted. As Figure 2.3 suggests, this could be a mistake.

The several sources of variation are cumulative. Figure 2.4 illustrates this for the measurement of blood pressure. Variation due to measurement contributes relatively little, although it covers as much as a 12 mm Hg range for the various observers. On the other hand, each patient's blood pressure does vary a great deal from moment to moment throughout the day, so that any single blood pressure reading might be quite unrepresentative of the usual for that patient. Much of this variation is not random: blood pressure is generally higher when people are awake, excited, visiting physicians, or taking over-the-counter "cold" medications. Of course, we are most interested in the bottom curve, to know how an individual's blood pressure compares to that of his or her peers.

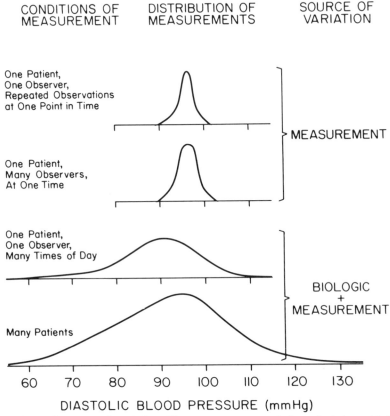

| CONDITIONS OF
MEASUREMENT | DISTRIBUTION OF
MEASUREMENTS | SOURCE OF
VARIATION |

One Patient,
One Observer,
Repeated Observations
at One Point in Time

One Patient,
Many Observers,
At One Time

MEASUREMENT

One Patient,
One Observer,
Many Times of Day

BIOLOGIC
+
MEASUREMENT

Many Patients

60   70   80   90   100   110   120   130

DIASTOLIC BLOOD PRESSURE (mmHg)

Figure 2.4.   Sources of variation. The measurement of diastolic (phase V) blood pressure. (Data from Fletcher RH, Fletcher SW, unpublished; and Boe J, Humerfelt S, Wedervang F, Oecon C: *Acta Med Scand* 321:5–313, 1957.)

Effects of Variation

Another way of thinking about variation is in terms of its net effect on the validity of a measurement and what can be done about it.

Random variation will, on the average, result in no net misrepresentation of the true state of the phenomenon. Inaccuracy due to random variation can be reduced by taking a larger sample of what is being measured—for example, counting more cells on a blood smear or examining a larger area of a urine sediment. Also, the extent of random variation can be estimated by means of inferential statistics (Chapter 9).

On the other hand, biased results are systematically different from the true value, no matter how many times they are repeated. For example, when investigating a patient suspected of having an infiltrative liver disease (perhaps because of an elevated serum alkaline phosphatase) a single liver biopsy may be subject to bias, depending on how the lesions are distributed in the liver. If the lesion is a metastasis in the left lobe of the liver a biopsy in the usual place (the right lobe) would be biased. On the other hand, a biopsy for miliary tuberculosis, which is represented by millions of small granulomata throughout the liver, would be inaccurate only through random variation. Similarly, all of the high values for VPDs shown in Figure 2.3 were recorded on the first day, and most of the low values on the third. The days were biased estimates of each other, because of variation in VPD rate from day to day.

DISTRIBUTIONS

Data that are measured on interval scales are often presented as a figure called a *frequency distribution* showing the number (or proportion) of a defined group of people possessing the different values of the measurement (Fig. 2.5). Presenting interval data as a frequency distribution conveys the information in relatively fine detail.

However, it is frequently convenient to summarize distributions even further. Indeed, summarization is imperative if a large number of distributions are to be presented and compared.

Two basic properties of distributions are used to summarize them. One

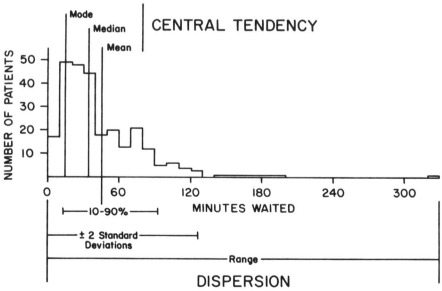

Figure 2.5. Measures of central tendency and dispersion. Patients' waiting time in a medical clinic. (Data from O'Malley MS, Fletcher SW, Fletcher RH, Earp JA: Measuring patient waiting time in a practice setting: a comparison of methods. *J Ambul Care Manage* 6:20–27, 1983.)

is *central tendency*, the middle of the distribution. The other is *dispersion*, how spread out the values are. Several ways of expressing central tendency and dispersion, along with their advantages and disadvantages, are illustrated in Figure 2.5 and summarized in Tables 2.3 and 2.4.

Actual Distributions

The frequency distributions of four common blood tests—potassium,

Table 2.3
Expressions of Central Tendency

EXPRESSION	DEFINITION	ADVANTAGES	DISADVANTAGES
Mean	Sum of values for observations / Number of observations	Well suited for mathematical manipulation	Affected by extreme values
Median	The point where the number of observations above equals the number below	Not easily influenced by extreme values	Not well suited for mathematical manipulation
Mode	Most frequently occurring value	Simplicity of meaning	Sometimes there are no, or many, most frequent values

Table 2.4
Expressions of Dispersion

EXPRESSION	DEFINITION	ADVANTAGES	DISADVANTAGES
Range	From lowest to highest value in a distribution	Includes all values	Greatly affected by extreme values
Standard deviation[a]	The absolute value of the average difference of individual values from the mean	Well suited for mathematical manipulation	For non-Gaussian distributions, does not describe a known proportion of the observations
Percentile, decile, quartile, etc.	The proportion of all observations falling between specified values	Describes the "unusualness" of a value without assumptions about the shape of a distribution	Not well suited for statistical manipulation

[a] $\sqrt{\dfrac{\Sigma(X - \bar{X})^2}{N - 1}}$

where: X = each observation
$\bar{X}$ = mean of all observations
N = number of observations

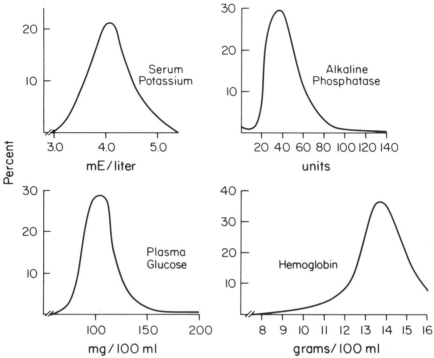

Figure 2.6. Examples of frequency distributions for clinical measurements. (Data from Martin HF, Gudzinowicz BJ, Fanger H: *Normal Values in Clinical Chemistry.* New York, Marcel Dekker, 1975.)

alkaline phosphatase, glucose, and hemoglobin—are shown in Figure 2.6. In general, most of the values appear in the middle of the distributions. The distributions are smooth, and except for the central part of the curves there are no "humps" or irregularities in the curves. The high and low ends of the distributions stretch out into tails, with the tail at one end often being more prominent than the tail at the other (i.e., the curves are "skewed" toward that end). Whereas some of the distributions are skewed toward higher values, others are skewed in the opposite direction. In other words, these distributions are unimodal and roughly bell-shaped, although asymmetric; otherwise they do not resemble each other.

The distribution of values for many laboratory tests changes with characteristics of the patients, such as age, sex, race, or nutrition. Therefore, what might be a perfectly ordinary value for one person could be unusual for another. Figure 2.7 shows how the distribution of one such test, blood urea nitrogen (BUN), changes with age. A BUN of 25 mg/100 ml would be unusually high for a young person, but not particularly remarkable for an older person.

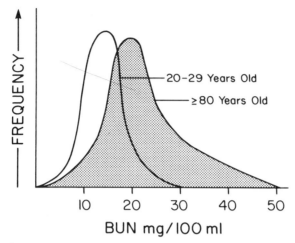

Figure 2.7. Change in normal function with age. BUN in people aged 20–29 and 80 or older. (Data from Martin HF, Gudzinowicz BJ, Fanger H: *Normal Values in Clinical Chemistry.* New York, Marcel Dekker, 1975.)

Normal Distribution

Another kind of distribution, called the normal or "Gaussian" distribution,[a] should be contrasted with naturally occurring distributions, inasmuch as the two are frequently equated. The normal curve describes the distribution of repeated measurements of the same physical object by the same instrument. Dispersion of values represents random variation alone. A normal curve is shown in Figure 2.8. The curve is symmetrical and bell shaped. It has the mathematical property that about two-thirds of the observations fall within 1 standard deviation of the mean, and about 95% within 2 standard deviations.

Although clinical distributions often resemble a normal distribution in that they are usually smooth, unimodal, and bell shaped, the resemblance is superficial. As one statistician put it (7):

... The experimental fact is that for most physiologic variables the distribution is smooth, unimodal, and skewed, and that mean ±2 standard deviations does not cut off the desired 95%. We have no mathematical, statistical, or other theorems that enable us to predict the shape of the distributions of physiologic measurements.

Whereas the normal distribution is derived from mathematical theory and reflects only random variation, many other sources of variation contribute to distributions of clinical measurements, particularly biologic differences among subjects. As a result, if distributions of clinical measure-

---

[a] The normal curve was first described by Johann Gauss, a German mathematician and physical scientist, in the 19th century.

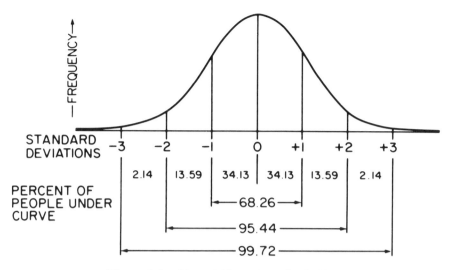

Figure 2.8.   Normal (Gaussian) distribution.

ments of many people resemble normal curves, it is largely by accident. However, it is often assumed, as a matter of convenience (because means and standard deviations are relatively easy to calculate and manipulate mathematically), that clinical measurements are normally distributed.

CRITERIA FOR ABNORMALITY

It would be convenient if the frequency distributions of measurements for normal and abnormal people were so distinct that they could be recognized as two populations on a frequency distribution. Figure 2.9, showing the activity of an enzyme that is inherited through a single gene, is an example of an actual distribution in which this is possible.

However, the distributions with which clinicians usually work do not display sharp breaks or two peaks that distinguish normal from abnormal results. There are several reasons why this is so. For many laboratory tests, there are not even theoretical reasons for believing that distinct populations—well and diseased—exist. Disease is acquired by degrees, and so there is a smooth transition from low to high values with increasing degrees of dysfunction. Laboratory tests reflecting organ failure, such as blood urea nitrogen for renal failure, behave in this way.

In other situations, well and diseased persons do in fact belong to separate populations. For example, frequency distributions of serum calciums for people with and without hyperparathyroidism would appear different. However, in unselected populations the diseased patients often do not stand out because there are very few of them relative to normal people and because laboratory values for the diseased population overlap

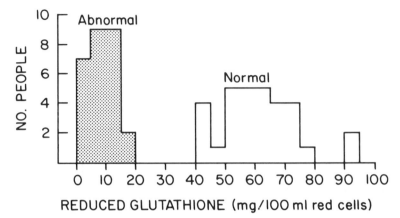

Figure 2.9. Clean separation of normal from abnormal people. Assay for reduced glutathione in male relatives of patients with glucose 6-phosphate dehydrogenase deficiency. (Redrawn from Childs B, Zinkham W, Browne EA, Kimbro EL, Torbert JV. A genetic study of a defect in glutathione metabolism of the erythrocyte. *Bull Johns Hopkins Hosp* 102:21–37, 1958.)

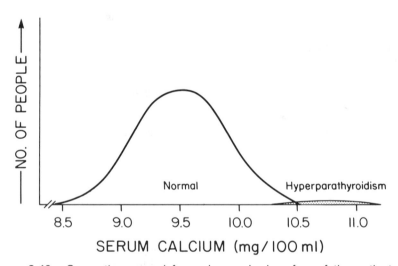

Figure 2.10. Separating normal from abnormal when few of the patients are abnormal. Hypothetical distribution of serum calciums in normal and hyperparathyroid people in the general population (prevalence of normal/prevalence of hyperparathyroid 200/1).

those for normals. The curve for diseased people is "swallowed up" by the larger curve for normal people (Fig. 2.10).

If, on the other hand, normal and diseased populations are mixed in more equal proportions—perhaps by selecting out for testing people with an unusually high likelihood of disease—then the resulting distribution could be truly bimodal. Even so, it would not be possible to choose a test value that clearly separates diseased and nondiseased persons (see Chapter 3).

If there is no sharp dividing line between normal and abnormal, and the clinician can choose where the line is placed, what ground rules should be used to decide? Three criteria have proven useful: being unusual, being sick, and being treatable. For a given measurement, these approaches bear no necessary relation to each other, so that what might be considered abnormal using one criterion might be normal by another.

Abnormal as Unusual

In clinical medicine, normal usually refers to the most frequently occurring or usual condition. Whatever occurs often is considered normal, and what occurs infrequently is abnormal. This is a statistical definition, based on the frequency of a characteristic in a defined, usually nondiseased population. The reference population need not be nondiseased. For example, we may say that it is normal to have pain after surgery or for middle-aged Americans to have serum cholesterols over 200 mg/dl.

It is tempting to be more specific by defining what is unusual in mathematical terms. One commonly used way of establishing a cutoff point between normal and abnormal is to agree, somewhat arbitrarily, that all values beyond 2 standard deviations from the mean are abnormal. On the assumption that the distribution in question approximates a normal (Gaussian) distribution, 2.5% of observations would then appear in each tail of a distribution and be considered abnormal.

Of course, as already pointed out, most biologic measurements are not normally distributed. So it is better to describe unusual values, whatever the proportion chosen, as percentiles of the underlying distribution. In this way, it is possible to make a direct statement about how infrequent a value is, without making assumptions about the shape of the distribution from which it came.

The statistical definition of normality serves adequately in some situations. But there are several ways in which it can be ambiguous or misleading.

1. If all values beyond an arbitrary statistical limit—for example, the 95th percentile—were considered abnormal, then the prevalence of all diseases would be the same, 5%. This is inconsistent with our usual way of thinking about disease frequency. There is no general relationship between the degree of statistical unusualness and clinical disease. The relationship depends on the disease in question. For some measurements, deviations from usual are associated with disease to an important degree only at quite extreme values, well beyond the 95th or even the 99th percentile.

Example—The World Health Organization considers anemia to be present when hemoglobin (Hb) levels are below 12 grams/100 ml in adult nonpregnant females.

In a British survey of women aged 20–64, Hb fell below 12 grams/100 ml for 11% of 920 nonpregnant women, twice as many as would be expected if ±2 standard deviations were the criterion for normality. But were they "diseased" in any way, by virtue of their low Hb? Two possibilities come to mind: The low Hb may be associated with symptoms; or it may be a marker for serious underlying disease. Symptoms like fatigue, dizziness, and irritability were not correlated with Hb level, at least for women whose Hb was above 8.0. Moreover, oral iron, given to women with Hb between 8.0 and 12.0, increased their Hb by an average of 2.30 grams/100 ml, but did not lead to any greater improvement in symptoms than was experienced by women given placebo. As for serious underlying disease, it is true that occasionally, low Hb may be a manifestation of cancer, chronic infection, or rheumatic diseases. But only a very small proportion of women with low Hb have these conditions.

Thus, only at Hb levels below 8.0, which occurred in less than 1% of these women, might anemia be an important health problem (8).

2. Many laboratory tests are related to risk of disease over their entire range of values, from low to high. Figure 2.11 illustrates how one such test, serum cholesterol, is related to the incidence of coronary heart disease. There is an almost threefold increase in risk from the "low normal" to the "high normal" range.

3. Some extreme values are distinctly unusual but preferable to more usual ones. This is particularly true at the low end of some distributions. Who would not be pleased to have a serum creatinine of 0.3 mg/100 ml or a systolic blood pressure of 100 mm Hg? Both are unusually low, but they represent better than average health or risk.

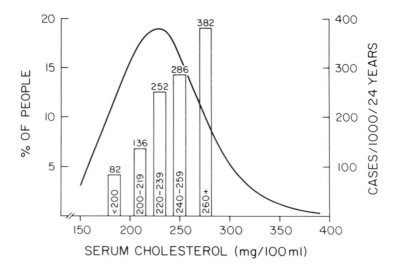

Figure 2.11. Increasing risk through the normal range. Serum cholesterol and the risk of coronary heart disease in men aged 30–39. (Adapted from Dawber TR: *The Framingham Study.* Cambridge, Harvard University Press, 1980.)

4. Sometimes patients are clearly diseased, even though laboratory tests diagnostic of their disease are in the usual range for healthy people. Examples include low pressure hydrocephalus, normal pressure glaucoma, and normocalcemic hyperparathyroidism.

Abnormal as Associated with Disease

A sounder approach to distinguishing normal from abnormal is to call abnormal those observations that are regularly associated with disease, disability, or death—that is, any clinically meaningful departure from good health. The disease may be expressed directly by symptoms, or predicted by characteristics that are themselves strongly associated with poor health, such as "risk factors" or clinically important physical signs. (This caveat is mentioned in order to avoid the kind of circular reasoning whereby statistically unusual measurements are called diseases, and the unusualness is then found to be a good predictor of disease.)

Judgments about what is an important risk may vary, even where the risk is known (Fig. 2.12). Most would agree that the risk of developing gout is negligible at uric acid levels below 7.0 mg/100 ml (this includes 95.2% of the population). After that, the risk starts to rise so that at levels greater than 9.0 many people develop gout. The decision as to where abnormality begins depends on a judgment about the level of risk worth preventing, given current methods. For serum uric acid, it is conventional to choose that value around 8.0 or 9.0 mg/100 ml.

Abnormal as Treatable

For some conditions, particularly those that are not troublesome in their own right (i.e., are asymptomatic), it is better to consider a measurement abnormal only if its treatment leads to a better outcome. This is because not everything that marks risk can be successfully treated. Removal of risk factors may not remove risk, either because the factor is not itself a cause of disease, but only related to a cause, or because irreversible damage has already occurred. Also, to label people as abnormal can cause adverse psychological effects that cannot be justified if treatment cannot improve the outlook.

What we consider treatable changes with time. At their best, therapeutic decisions are grounded on evidence in the form of well-conducted clinical trials (Chapter 8). As new knowledge accumulates from the results of clinical trials, the level at which treatment is considered useful may change. Figure 2.13 shows how accumulating evidence for treating hypertension has changed our definition of what level is treatable. With the passage of time, successively lower levels of diastolic blood pressure have been shown to be worth treating.

REGRESSION TO THE MEAN

When clinicians encounter an unexpectedly abnormal test result, they

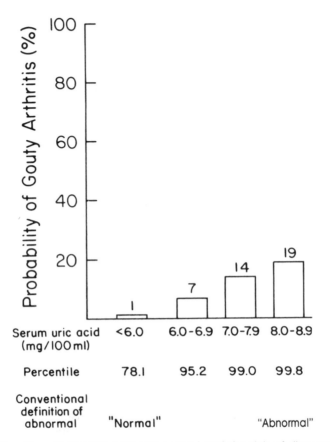

Figure 2.12. The relationship between normal and the risk of disease. The risk for men of having gouty arthritis at various levels of serum uric acid. (Data from Hall AP, Barry PE, Dawber TR, McNamara PM. Epidemiology of gout and hyperuricemia. A long term population study. *Am J Med* 42:27–37, 1967.)

tend to repeat it. Often the second test result is closer to normal. Why does this happen? Should it be reassuring?

Patients selected because they represent an extreme value in a distribution can be expected, on the average, to have less extreme values on subsequent measurements. This can occur for purely statistical reasons (random variation) and is called *regression to the mean.*

Example—In a trial of the effect of reducing multiple risk factors on the subsequent incidence of coronary heart disease, (The Multiple Risk Factor Intervention Trial), high-risk patients were selected for study. Elevated blood pressure was one of the risk factors that caused people to be considered for the study. People

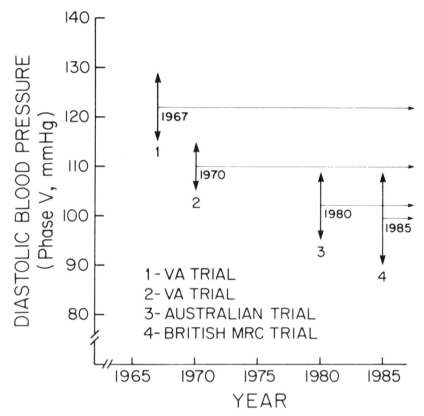

Figure 2.13. The changing definition of treatable disease. Accumulating evidence for treating successively lower levels of blood pressure. (Data from Veterans Administration Cooperative Study Group on Antihypertensive Agents: *JAMA* 202:1028–1034, 1967; Veterans Administration Cooperative Study Group on Hypertensive Agents. *JAMA* 213:1143–1152, 1970; Management committee; Australian therapeutic trial of mild hypertension. *Lancet* 1:1261–1267, 1980; and Medical Research Council Working Party: MRC trial of treatment of mild hypertension: principal results. *Br Med J* 291:97–104, 1985.)

were screened for inclusion in the study on three consecutive visits. Blood pressures at those visits, before any therapeutic interventions were undertaken, were as follows:

Visit	Mean Diastolic Blood Pressure (mm Hg)
1	99.2
2	91.2
3	90.7

There was a substantial fall in mean blood pressure between the first and the third visits. The authors attributed this fall to regression to the mean, as well as to a tendency for patients to be more relaxed on later visits. (There was also a fall in serum cholesterol, which presumably was not affected by moment-to-moment anxiety (9).)

Regression to the mean arose in the following way. People were first selected because their initial blood pressure fell above an arbitrarily selected cutoff point in the tail of a distribution of blood pressures for all the patients examined. Some of those people would remain above the cutoff point on subsequent measurements because their true blood pressures were ordinarily higher than average. But others who were found to have blood pressures above the cutoff point during the initial screening usually had lower pressure readings. They were included only because they happened, through random variation, to have high blood pressures at that point in time. When their blood pressures were retaken they had lower values than on the first visit. This tended to drag downward the mean blood pressure of the subgroup originally found to have readings above the cutoff point.

Thus, patients who are singled out from others because they possess a laboratory test that is unusually high or low can be expected, on the average, to be closer to the center of the distribution if the test is repeated. Moreover, subsequent values are likely to be more accurate estimates of the true value, which could be obtained if the measurement were repeated for a particular patient many times. So the time-honored practice of repeating laboratory tests that are found to be abnormal and calling the second one, which is often within normal limits, the correct one is not just wishful thinking. It has a sound theoretical basis. It also has an empirical basis. For example, it has been shown that half of serum T_4 tests found to be outside normal limits on screening were within normal limits when repeated (10). However, the more extreme the initial reading is, the less likely it is to be normal if it is repeated.

SUMMARY

Clinical phenomena are measured on nominal, ordinal, and interval scales. Although many clinical observations fall on a continuum of values, for practical reasons they are often simplified into dichotomous (present/absent) categories. Observations of clinical phenomena vary because of measurement error, differences in individuals from time to time, and differences among individuals. The performance of a method of measurement, the extent to which it correctly classifies, is expressed in terms of validity (does it measure what it intends to measure?) and reliability (do repeated measures of the same thing give the same result?).

Frequency distributions for clinical variables have different shapes; they can be summarized by describing their central tendency and dispersion.

Laboratory values from normal and abnormal people often overlap. Choice of a point at which normal ends and abnormal begins is arbitrary and often related to one of three definitions of abnormality: statistically unusual, associated with disease, or treatable. If patients with extreme values of a test are selected and the test is repeated, the second value is likely to fall closer to the central (statistically normal) part of the frequency distribution, a phenomenon called regression to the mean.

REFERENCES

1. Afifi AA, Clark V: *Computer-aided Multivariate Analysis.* Belmont, CA, Lifetime Learning, 1984.
2. Colton T: *Statistics in Medicine.* Boston, Little, Brown and Co, 1974.
3. Feinstein AR: *Clinical Epidemiology. The Architecture of Clinical Research.* Philadelphia, WB Saunders, 1985.
4. Feinstein AR: The need for humanized science in evaluating medication. *Lancet* 2:421–423, 1972.
5. Day E, Maddern L, Wood C: Auscultation of foetal heart rate: an assessment of its error and significance. *Br Med J* 4:422–424, 1968.
6. Morganroth J, Michelson EL, Horowitz LN, Josephson ME, Pearlman AS, Dunkman WB: Limitations of routine long-term electrocardiographic monitoring to assess ventricular ectopic frequency. *Circulation* 58:408–414, 1978.
7. Elveback LR, Guillier CL, Keating FR: Health, normality, and the ghost of Gauss. *JAMA* 211:69–75, 1970.
8. Elwood PC, Waters WE, Greene WJW, Sweetnam P: Symptoms and circulating hemoglobin level. *J Chron Dis* 21:615–628, 1969.
9. Kuller L, Neaton J, Caggiula A, Falvao-Gerard L: Primary prevention of heart attacks: The multiple risk factor intervention trial. *Am J Epidemiol* 112:185–199, 1980.
10. Epstein KA, Schneiderman LJ, Bush JW, Zettner A: The "abnormal" screening serum thyroxine (T_4): Analysis of physician response, outcome, cost and health effectiveness. *J Chron Dis* 34:175–190, 1981.

SUGGESTED READINGS

Department of Clinical Epidemiology and Biostatistics, McMaster University: Clinical disagreement I. How often it occurs and why. *Can Med Assoc J* 123:499–504, 1980.
Department of Clinical Epidemiology and Biostatistics, McMaster University: Clinical disagreement II. How to avoid it and how to learn from one's mistakes. *Can Med Assoc J* 123:613–617, 1980.
Feinstein AR: *Clinical Judgment.* Baltimore, Williams & Wilkins, 1967.
Feinstein AR: *Section 3. Problems in Measurement, Clinical Biostatistics,* St. Louis, CV Mosby, 1977.
Galen RS, Gambino SR: *Beyond Normality. The Predictive Value and Efficacy of Medical Diagnosis.* New York, John Wiley & Sons, 1975.
Koran LM: The reliability of clinical methods, data and judgment. *N Engl J Med* 293:642–646, 695–701, 1975.
Mainland D: Remarks on clinical "norms." *Clin Chem* 17:267–274, 1971.

chapter **3**

DIAGNOSIS

APPEARANCES to the mind are of four kinds.
Things either are what they appear to be;
or they neither are, nor appear to be;
or they are, and do not appear to be;
or they are not, yet appear to be.
Rightly to aim in all these cases
is the wise man's task.—*Epictetus*
2nd CENTURY AD (1)

Clinicians devote a great deal of time to determining diagnoses for complaints or abnormalities presented by their patients; they arrive at the diagnoses after applying various diagnostic tests. Even so, few practicing physicians receive formal training in the interpretation of diagnostic tests. Most competent clinicians use good judgment, a thorough knowledge of the literature, and a kind of rough-and-ready approach to how the information should be organized. However, there are also basic principles with which a clinician should be familiar when interpreting diagnostic tests. This chapter will deal with those principles.

A "diagnostic test" ordinarily is taken to mean a test performed in a laboratory. But the principles to be discussed in this chapter apply equally well to clinical information obtained from history, physical examination, or x-rays. They also apply where a constellation of findings serves as a diagnostic test. Thus, one might speak of the value of arthritis, carditis, and chorea in diagnosing rheumatic fever or of hemoptysis and weight loss in a cigarette smoker as indicators of lung cancer.

SIMPLIFYING DATA

In the previous chapter, it was pointed out that clinical measurements, including data from diagnostic tests, are expressed on nominal, ordinal, or interval scales. Regardless of the kind of data produced by diagnostic tests, clinicians are inclined to reduce the data to a simpler form in order to make it useful in practice. Most ordinal scales are examples of this simplification process. Obviously, heart murmurs can vary from very loud to inaudible. But expressing subtle gradations in the intensity of murmurs is both tedious and unnecessary. A simple ordinal scale, grade I to VI, serves just as well. More often, complex data are reduced to a simple dichotomy—for example, present/absent, abnormal/normal, or diseased/well. This is particularly so when test results are used to decide on treatment. At any given point in time, therapeutic decisions are either/or decisions. Either treatment is begun or it is withheld.

The use of blood pressure data to decide about therapy is an example of how we simplify information for practical purposes. Blood pressure is ordinarily measured to the nearest millimeter of mercury—that is, on an interval scale. However, most physicians choose a particular level (e.g., 90 mm Hg diastolic pressure) at which they initiate treatment. In doing so, they have transformed interval into nominal (in this case, dichotomous) data. To take the example further, it may be that a physician would choose a treatment plan according to whether the patient's diastolic blood pressure is "mildly elevated" (90–104 mm Hg), "moderately elevated" (105–114 mm Hg), or "severely elevated" (115 mm Hg and above). The doctor would then be reacting to the test in an ordinal manner.

THE ACCURACY OF A TEST RESULT

As all clinicians quickly learn, establishing diagnoses is an imperfect process, resulting in a probability rather than a certainty of being right. That being the case, it behooves the clinician to become familiar with the mathematical relationships between the properties of diagnostic tests and the information they yield in various clinical situations. In many instances, understanding these issues will help the clinician resolve some uncertainty surrounding the use of diagnostic tests. In other situations, it may only increase understanding of the uncertainty. Occasionally, it may convince the clinician to increase his or her level of uncertainty!

A simple way of looking at the relationships between a test's results and the true diagnosis is shown in Figure 3.1. The test is considered to be either positive (abnormal) or negative (normal) and the disease either present or absent. There are then four possible interpretations of test results, two of which are correct and two wrong. The test has given the correct answer when it is positive in the presence of disease or negative in the absence of the disease. On the other hand, the test has been misleading if it is positive when the disease is absent (false positive) or negative when the disease is present (false negative).

The "Gold Standard"

Assessment of the test's accuracy rests on its relationship to some way of knowing whether the disease is truly present or not—a sound assessment

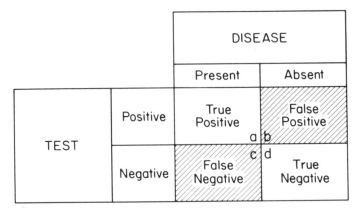

Figure 3.1.   The relationship between a diagnostic test result and the occurrence of disease. There are two possibilities for the test result to be correct (true positive and true negative) and two possibilities for the result to be incorrect (false positive and false negative).

of the truth. As it turns out, this gold standard is often elusive. Sometimes the standard of accuracy is itself a relatively simple and inexpensive test, such as a throat culture for Group A β-hemolytic streptococcus to validate the clinical impression of strep throat. However, this is usually not the case. More often, one must turn to relatively elaborate, expensive, or risky tests in order to be certain whether the disease is present or absent. Among these are tissue diagnoses, radiologic contrast procedures, prolonged follow-up—and, of course, autopsies.

Because it is almost always more costly, and sometimes less feasible, to use these more accurate ways of establishing the truth, simpler tests are often substituted for the rigorous gold standard, at least initially. Chest x-rays and sputum smears are used to determine the nature of pneumonia, rather than lung biopsy with examination of the diseased lung tissue. Similarly, electrocardiograms and serum enzymes are ordinarily used to establish the diagnosis of acute myocardial infarction, rather than biopsy. The simpler tests are used as proxies for more elaborate but more accurate ways of establishing the presence of disease with the understanding that some risk of misclassification results, which is justified by the feasibility of the simpler tests.

It would be helpful if our commonly used diagnostic tests were all backed by sound data comparing their accuracy to an appropriate standard. The goal of all clinical studies describing the value of diagnostic tests should be to obtain data for all four of the cells in Figure 3.1. Without all these data, it is not possible to answer important questions about the performance of the tests.

Lack of Information on Negative Tests

Given that the goal is to fill in all of the four cells, it must be stated that sometimes this is difficult to do in the real world. It may be that an objective and valid means of establishing the diagnosis exists, but is not available for the purposes of formally establishing the properties of a diagnostic test for ethical or practical reasons. Consider the situation in which most information about diagnostic tests is obtained. Published accounts come primarily from clinical, and not research, settings. Under these circumstances, physicians are using the test in the process of caring for patients. They ordinarily feel justified in proceeding with more exhaustive evaluation, in the patient's best interest, only when preliminary diagnostic tests are positive. They are naturally reluctant to initiate an aggressive workup, with its associated risk and expense, when the test is negative. As a result, information on negative tests, whether true negative or false negative, tends to be much less complete in the medical literature.

This problem is illustrated by a study of the relative merits of two tests for diagnosing gallstones—ultrasonic cholecystography and an older, conventional test, radiographic oral cholecystography (2). If patients had abnormal radiographic oral cholecystograms, they were submitted to surgery where the true diagnosis of gallstones could be confirmed or rejected. However, patients with normal oral cholecystograms were not sent to surgery, whether or not ultrasound indicated stones. The authors understandably considered it unethical to submit patients to surgery on the basis of a new and unproven test. Nevertheless, the situation leaves us unable to determine the false negative rate for oral cholecystograms or for any of the ultrasound results that were accompanied by a negative oral cholecystogram.

For diseases that are not self-limited, and ordinarily become overt in a matter of a few years after they are first suspected, the results of followup can serve as a gold standard. Most cancers and chronic, degenerative diseases fall into this category. For them, validation is possible even if on-the-spot confirmation of a test's performance is not feasible because the immediately available gold standard is too risky, involved, or expensive. All it takes is time and patience.

Lack of Objective Standards for Disease

For some conditions, there are simply no hard and fast criteria for diagnosis. Angina pectoris is one of these. The clinical manifestations were described nearly a century ago and are familiar to all medical students and many laymen as well. Yet there is still no better way to substantiate the presence of angina pectoris than a carefully taken history. Certainly a great many objectively measurable phenomena are related to this clinical syndrome—for example, the presence of coronary lesions seen on angiography, increased concentrations of lactate in coronary sinus blood, and characteristic abnormalities on electrocardiograms both at rest and with exercise. All are more commonly found in patients believed to have angina pectoris. But none is so uniquely tied to the clinical syndrome that it will serve as the standard by which the condition is considered present or absent.

Sometimes, usually in an effort to be "rigorous," circular reasoning is applied. The validity of a laboratory test is established by comparing its results to a clinical diagnosis, based on a careful history of symptoms and a physical examination. Once established, the test is then used to validate the clinical diagnosis gained from history and physical examination! An example would be the use of manometry to "confirm" irritable bowel syndrome, because the contraction pattern demonstrated by manometry and believed to be characteristic of irritable bowel was validated by clinical impression in the first place.

Consequences of Imperfect Standards

Because of such difficulties as these, it is frequently not possible for physicians in practice to find information on how well the tests they use compare to a thoroughly trustworthy standard. They must choose as their standard of validity another test that admittedly is imperfect but is considered the best available. This may force them into comparing one weak test against another, with one being taken as a standard of validity because it has had longer use or is considered superior by a consensus of experts. In doing so, a paradox may arise. If a new test is compared with an old (but inaccurate) standard test, the new test may seem worse even when it is actually better. For example, if the new test is more sensitive than the standard test, the additional patients identified by the new test would be considered false positives in relation to the old test. Just such a situation occurred in a comparison of real-time ultrasonography and oral cholecystography for the detection of gallstones (3). In five patients, ultrasound was positive for stones that were missed on an adequate cholecystogram. Two of the patients later underwent surgery and gallstones were found, so that for at least those two patients, the standard oral cholecystogram was actually less accurate than the newer real-time ultrasound. Similarly, if the new test is more often negative in patients who really do not have the disease, results for those patients will be considered false negatives compared to the old test. Thus, if an inaccurate standard of validity is used, a new test can perform no better than that standard and will seem inferior when it approximates the truth more closely.

SENSITIVITY AND SPECIFICITY

Figure 3.2 summarizes some relationships between a diagnostic test and the actual presence of disease. It is an expansion of Figure 3.1, with the addition of some useful definitions. Most of the rest of this chapter will deal with these relationships in detail. They are illustrated in Figure 3.3: The diagnostic test is housestaff's clinical impression of whether patients complaining of pharyngitis have a Group A β-hemolytic streptococcus infection or not, and the gold standard is a throat culture.

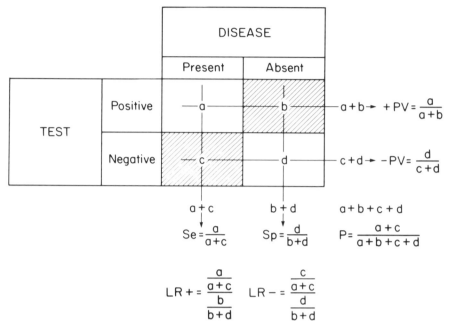

Figure 3.2.   Diagnostic test characteristics and definitions.

Definitions

As can be seen in Figure 3.2 *sensitivity* is defined as the proportion of people with the disease who have a positive test for the disease. A sensitive test will rarely miss people with the disease. *Specificity* is the proportion of people without the disease who have a negative test. A specific test will rarely misclassify people without the disease as diseased.

Applying these definitions to the pharyngitis example, 37 of the 149 patients with sore throats had positive cultures, and housestaff correctly diagnosed 27 of these—for a sensitivity of 73%. On the other hand, 112 patients had negative culture results; housestaff correctly withheld antibiotics from 77, for a specificity of 69%.

Uses of Sensitive Tests

Clinicians should take the sensitivity and specificity of a diagnostic test into account when a test is selected. A sensitive test (i.e., one that is usually positive in the presence of disease) should be chosen when there is an important penalty for missing a disease. This would be so, for example, when there is reason to suspect a dangerous but treatable condition, such as tuberculosis, syphilis, or Hodgkin's disease. Sensitive tests are also helpful during the early stages of a diagnostic workup when a great many possibilities are being considered, in order to reduce the number of possi-

		GROUP A β-HEMOLYTIC STREPTOCOCCUS ON THROAT CULTURE			
		Present	Absent		
CLINICAL DIAGNOSIS OF STREP PHARYNGITIS	Yes	27	35	62	$+PV = \dfrac{27}{62} = 44\%$
	No	10	77	87	$-PV = \dfrac{77}{87} = 88\%$
		37	112	149	

$$Se = \frac{27}{37} = 73\% \quad Sp = \frac{77}{112} = 69\% \quad P = \frac{37}{149} = 25\%$$

$$LR+ = \frac{\dfrac{27}{27+10}}{\dfrac{35}{35+77}} = 2.3 \quad LR- = \frac{\dfrac{10}{10+27}}{\dfrac{77}{77+35}} = .39$$

Figure 3.3. The accuracy of the clinical diagnosis of streptococcal pharyngitis compared to the results of throat culture. (Data from Fletcher SW, Hamann C: Emergency room management of patients with sore throats in a teaching hospital; influence of non-physician factors. *J Comm Health* 1:196–204, 1976.)

bilities. Diagnostic tests are used in these situations to "rule out" diseases— that is, to establish that certain diseases are unlikely possibilities. For example, one might choose a tuberculin skin test early in the evaluation of lung infiltrates because this test is usually positive in people with active tuberculosis. Finally, sensitive tests are useful when the probability of disease is relatively low and the purpose of the test is to discover disease. This is the case when the test is used to screen people without complaints, as in the periodic health examination (discussed in Chapter 8). In sum, a sensitive test is most helpful to the clinician when the test result is negative.

Uses of Specific Tests

Specific tests are useful to confirm (or "rule in") a diagnosis that has been suggested by other data. This is because a highly specific test is rarely positive in the absence of disease—that is, it gives few false positive results. Highly specific tests are particularly needed when false positive results can harm the patient physically, emotionally, or financially. Thus, before patients are subjected to cancer chemotherapy, with all its attendant risks, emotional trauma, and financial costs, tissue diagnosis is generally required instead of relying upon less specific tests. In sum, a specific test is most helpful when the test result is positive.

Trade-Offs between Sensitivity and Specificity

Generally there is a trade-off between the sensitivity and specificity of a diagnostic test. It is obviously desirable to have a test that is both highly sensitive and highly specific. Unfortunately, this is usually not possible.

A trade-off between sensitivity and specificity is required when clinical data take on a range of values. In those situations, the location of a *cut-off point*, the point on the continuum between normal and abnormal, is an arbitrary decision. As a consequence, for any given test result expressed on an interval scale, one characteristic (e.g., sensitivity) can only be increased at the expense of the other (e.g., specificity). Table 3.1 demonstrates this interrelationship for the diagnosis of diabetes. If we require that a blood sugar taken 2 hours after eating be greater than 180 mg% to diagnose diabetes, all of the people diagnosed as "diabetic" would certainly have the disease, but many other people with diabetes would be missed using this extremely demanding definition of the disease. The test would be very specific at the expense of sensitivity. At the other extreme, if anyone with a blood sugar of greater than 70 mg% were diagnosed as diabetic, very few people with the disease would be missed, but most normal people would be falsely labeled as having diabetes. The test would then be very sensitive but nonspecific. There is no way, using a single blood sugar determination under standard conditions, that one can improve both the sensitivity and specificity of the test at the same time.

Another way to express the relationship between sensitivity and specificity for a given test is to construct a curve, called a *receiver operator characteristic (ROC) curve*. An ROC curve for the use of a single blood

Table 3.1
Trade-Off between Sensitivity and Specificity when Diagnosing Diabetes[a]

BLOOD SUGAR LEVEL 2 HOURS AFTER EATING	SENSITIVITY	SPECIFICITY
mg/100 ml	%	%
70	98.6	8.8
80	97.1	25.5
90	94.3	47.6
100	88.6	69.8
110	85.7	84.1
120	71.4	92.5
130	64.3	96.9
140	57.1	99.4
150	50.0	99.6
160	47.1	99.8
170	42.9	100.0
180	38.6	100.0
190	34.3	100.0
200	27.1	100.0

[a] From *Diabetes Program Guide*, Public Health Service Publication No. 506, 1960.

sugar determination to diagnose diabetes mellitus is illustrated in Figure 3.4. It is constructed by plotting the true positive rate (sensitivity) against the false positive rate (1 − specificity). The values on the axes run from a probability of 0 to 1.0 (or, alternatively, from 0 to 100%).

Tests that discriminate well crowd toward the upper left corner of the ROC curve; for them, as the sensitivity is progressively lowered (the cut-off point is lowered) there is little or no loss in specificity until high levels of sensitivity are achieved. Tests that perform less well have curves that fall closer to the diagonal running from lower left to upper right, the line describing a test that contributes no information.

The ROC curve is used to describe the accuracy of a test over a range of cut-off points. It can serve as a nomogram for reading off the specificity that corresponds to a given sensitivity. It shows how severe the trade-off between sensitivity and specificity is for a test and can be used to help decide where the best cut-off point would be. The overall accuracy of a test can be described as the area under the ROC curve; the larger the area, the better the test.

Although clinicians are forced to make a trade-off between sensitivity and specificity for any given test, it is possible that a new test can be both more sensitive and more specific than its predecessors. Figure 3.5 compares the ROC curves for two tests used to diagnose brain tumors—computed tomography and radionuclide scanning. Computed tomography is both more sensitive and more specific than the older "brain scan."

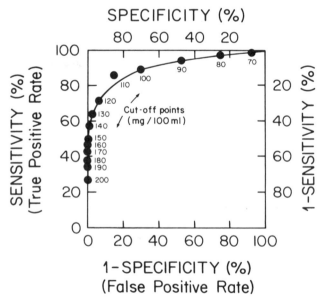

Figure 3.4. A receiver operator characteristic (ROC) curve. The accuracy of 2-hour postprandial blood sugar as a diagnostic test for diabetes mellitus. (Data from *Diabetes Program Guide*, Public Health Service Publication No. 506, 1960.)

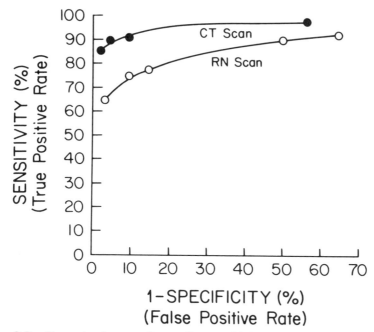

Figure 3.5. Example of a new diagnostic test with higher sensitivity and specificity than the older test. ROC curve for computed tomography (CT) and radionuclide scanning (RN) in diagnosing brain tumors. (In this figure, the cut-off points represent degrees of certainty about the diagnosis on the part of the radiologist, rather than numerical test values as in the previous examples. Redrawn from Griner PF, Mayewski RJ, Mushlin AI, Greenland P: Selection and interpretation of diagnostic tests and procedures. Principles and applications. *Ann Intern Med* 94:553–600, 1981.)

Obviously, tests that are both sensitive and specific are highly sought after and can be of enormous value. However, practicing clinicians rarely work with tests that are both highly sensitive and specific. So for the present, we must use other means for circumventing the trade-off between sensitivity and specificity. The most common way is to use the results of several tests together (see below).

ESTABLISHING SENSITIVITY AND SPECIFICITY

Not infrequently, a new diagnostic test is described in glowing terms when first introduced, only to be found wanting later when more experience with it has accumulated. Enthusiasm for the clinical value of serum carcinoembryonic antigen (CEA) waxed and then waned in this way. At first, CEA was considered a very promising means of diagnosing colon cancer. But CEA subsequently was shown to be increased in a wide variety of other malignancies, as well as in approximately 20% of smokers without cancer. This kind of confusion—initial enthusiasm followed by disappointment—arises not from any dishonesty on the part of early investigators or unfair skepticism by the medical community. Rather, it is related to misunderstandings—by the investigators, the readers, or both—about how the properties of diagnostic tests are established.

At the crudest level, the properties of a diagnostic test may be inaccurately described because an improper standard of validity has been chosen, as discussed previously. However, two other issues related to the selection of diseased and nondiseased patients can profoundly affect the determination of sensitivity and specificity as well. They are the spectrum of patients to which the test is applied, and bias in judging the test's performance. A third problem that can lead to inaccurate estimates of sensitivity and specificity is chance.

Spectrum of Patients

Difficulties may arise when patients used to describe the test's properties are different from those to whom the test will be applied in clinical practice. Early reports of a test often assess its value among persons who are clearly diseased as compared to persons who are clearly not diseased. The test may be able to distinguish between these extremes very well. But patients with the disease in question can differ in severity, stage, or duration of the disease, and the test's sensitivity/specificity may be higher in more severely affected patients. Similarly, some kinds of people without disease, such as these in whom disease is suspected, may have other conditions that cause a positive test, thereby increasing the false positive rate and decreasing specificity.

Example—Figure 3.6 illustrates how the performance of the test serum carcinoembryonic antigen (CEA) varies with the stage of colorectal cancer. CEA performs well for metastatic disease and poorly for localized cancer. Thus, the sensitivity and specificity for "colorectal cancer" would depend on the particular mix of stages of patients with disease used to describe the test, and its accuracy is more stable within stages.

In theory, sensitivity/specificity of a test are said to be independent of prevalence. (Work with Figure 3.2 to confirm this for yourself.) In practice, however, several characteristics of patients, such as stage and severity of disease, may be related both to the sensitivity/specificity of a test and to prevalence, because different kinds of patients are found in high- and low-prevalence situations.

Bias

Sometimes the sensitivity and specificity of a test are not established independently of the means by which the true diagnosis is established, leading to a biased assessment of its properties. This may occur in several ways.

As already pointed out, if the test is evaluated using data obtained during the course of a clinical evaluation of patients suspected of having the

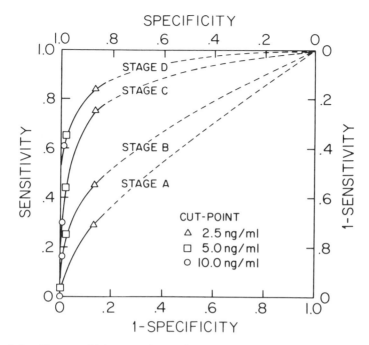

Figure 3.6. The sensitivity/specificity of a test varies with the stage of disease. ROC curve for carcinoembryonic antigen (CEA) as a diagnostic test for colorectal cancer according to stage of disease. (Redrawn from Fletcher RH: Carcinoembryonic antigen. *Ann Intern Med* 104:66–73, 1986.)

disease in question, a positive test may prompt the clinician to continue pursuing the diagnosis, increasing the likelihood that the disease will be found. On the other hand, a negative test may cause the clinician to abandon further testing, making it more likely that the disease, if present, will be missed. In other situations, the test result may be part of the information used to establish the diagnosis; or, conversely, the results of the test may be interpreted taking other clinical information or the final diagnosis into account.

Radiologists are frequently subject to this kind of bias when they read x-rays. Because x-ray interpretation is somewhat subjective, it is easy to be influenced by the clinical information provided. All clinicians experience the situation of having x-rays over-read because of a clinical impression, or conversely, going back over old x-rays in which a finding was missed because a clinical event was not known at the time and, therefore, attention was not directed to the particular area in the x-ray. Because of these biases, some radiologists prefer to read x-rays twice, first without and then with the clinical information.

All of these biases tend to increase the agreement between the test and the standard of validity. That is, they tend to make the test seem more useful than it actually is.

Chance

Values for sensitivity/specificity (or another characteristic of diagnostic tests, likelihood ratios, discussed below) are usually estimated from observations on relatively small samples of people with and without the disease of interest. Because of chance (random variation), in any one sample—particularly if it is small—the true sensitivity and specificity of the test can be misrepresented, even if there is no bias in the study. The particular values observed are compatible with a range of true values, typically characterized by the "95% confidence intervals"[a] (see Chapter 9). The width of this range of values defines the degree of precision of the estimates of sensitivity and specificity. Therefore, reported values for sensitivity and specificity should not be taken too literally.

Figure 3.7 shows how the precision of estimates of sensitivity increases as the number of people on which the estimate is based increases. In this particular example, the observed sensitivity of the diagnostic test is 75%. Figure 3.7 shows that if this estimate is based on only a few patients, by chance alone the true sensitivity could be as low as 45% and as high as nearly 100%. When more patients are studied, the 95% confidence interval narrows—that is, the precision of the estimate increases.

PREDICTIVE VALUE

As noted previously, sensitivity and specificity are properties of a test that are taken into account when a decision is made whether or not to order the test. But once the results of a diagnostic test are available, whether positive or negative, the sensitivity and specificity of the test are no longer of primary importance. This is because these values give the probability that a test will be positive or negative in persons known to have or not to have the disease. But if one knew the disease status of the patient, it would not be necessary to order the test! For the clinician, the dilemma is to determine whether or not the patient has the disease, given the results of a test.

---

[a] The 95% confidence interval of a proportion is easily estimated by the following formula, based on the binomial theorem:

$$p \pm 2^* \sqrt{\frac{p\,(1-p)}{N}}$$

where p = observed proportion
N = number of people observed

* More exactly, 1.96

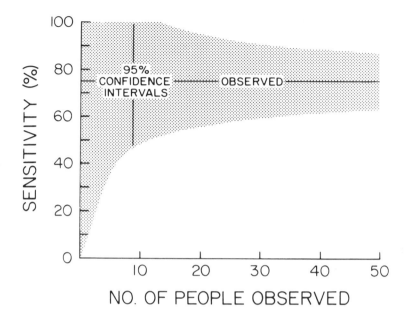

Figure 3.7. The precision of an estimate of sensitivity. The 95% confidence interval for an observed sensitivity of 75%, according to the number of people observed.

Definitions

The probability of disease, given the results of a test, is called the *predictive value* of the test (Fig. 3.2). Positive predictive value is the probability of disease in a patient with a positive (abnormal) test result. Negative predictive value is the probability of *not* having the disease when the test result is negative (normal). Predictive value is an answer to the question: If my patient's test result is positive (negative) what are the chances that my patient does (does not) have the disease? Predictive value is sometimes called *posterior* (or *posttest*) probability. Figure 3.3 illustrates these concepts. Among the patients treated with antibiotics for streptococcal pharyngitis, less than one-half (44%) had the condition by culture (positive predictive value). The negative predictive value of the housestaff's diagnostic impressions was better; of the 87 patients thought not to have streptococcal pharyngitis, the impression was correct for 77 (88%).

Terms summarizing the overall value of a test have been described. One such term, *accuracy*, is the proportion of all test results, both positive and negative, that are correct. (For the pharyngitis example in Figure 3.3, the accuracy of housestaff's diagnostic impressions was 70%.) In most cases, however, this summary term is too crude to be useful clinically because specific information about the component parts—which is what doctors need—is lost when they are aggregated into a single index.

Determinants of Predictive Value

The predictive value of a test is not a property of the test alone. It is determined by the sensitivity and specificity of the test and the prevalence of disease in the population being tested,[b] where prevalence has its customary meaning—the proportion of persons in a defined population at a given point in time with the condition in question. Prevalence is also called *prior* (or *pretest*) *probability*. (For a full discussion of prevalence, see Chapter 4.)

As evident in Figure 3.2, the more sensitive a test is, the better will be its negative predictive value (the more confident the clinician can be that a patient with a negative test result does not have the disease being sought). Conversely, the more specific the test is, the better will be its positive predictive value.

Because predictive value is also influenced by prevalence, it is not independent of the setting in which the test is used. Positive results even for a very specific test, when applied to patients with a low likelihood of having the disease, will be largely false positives. Similarly, negative results, even for a very sensitive test, when applied to patients with a high chance of having the disease, are likely to be false negatives. In sum, the interpretation of a positive or negative diagnostic test result should vary from setting to setting, according to estimated prevalence of disease in the particular setting.

This principle is not intuitively obvious. For those who are skeptical it might help to consider how a test would perform at the extremes of prevalence. Remember that no matter how sensitive and specific a test might be (short of perfection), there will still be a small proportion of patients who are misclassified by it. Imagine a population in which no one has the disease. In such a group all positive results, even for a very specific test, will be false positives. Therefore, as the prevalence of disease in a population approaches zero, the positive predictive value of a test also approaches zero. Conversely, if everyone in a population tested has the disease, all negative results will be false negatives, even for a very sensitive test. As prevalence approaches 100%, negative predictive value approaches zero. Another way for the skeptic to convince him- or herself of these relationships is to work with the table in Figure 3.3, holding sensitivity and specificity constant, changing prevalence, and calculating the resulting predictive values.

The effect of prevalence on positive predictive value, for a test with high sensitivity and specificity, is illustrated in Figure 3.8. When prevalence of disease in the population tested is relatively high—over several percent—

---

[b] The mathematical formula relating sensitivity, specificity, and prevalence to positive predictive value is derived from Bayes' theorem of conditional probabilities:

$$\text{Positive predictive value} = \frac{\text{Sensitivity} \times \text{prevalence}}{(\text{Sensitivity} \times \text{prevalence}) + (1 - \text{specificity}) \times (1 - \text{prevalence})}$$

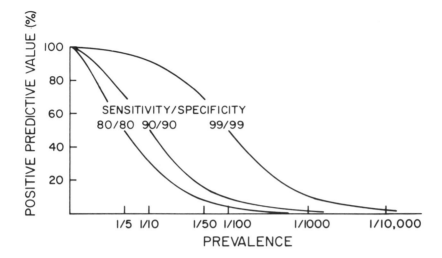

Figure 3.8. Positive predictive value according to sensitivity, specificity, and prevalence of disease.

Table 3.2
Effect of Prevalence on Predictive Value: Positive Predictive Value of Prostatic Acid Phosphatase for Prostatic Cancer (Sensitivity = 70%, Specificity = 90%) in Various Clinical Settings[a]

SETTING	PREVALENCE	POSITIVE PREDICTIVE VALUE
	cases/100,000	%
General population	35	0.4
Men, age 75 or greater	500	5.6
Clinically suspicious prostatic nodule	50,000	93.0

[a] From Watson RA, Tang DB: The predictive value of prostatic acid phosphatase as a screening test for prostatic cancer. *N Engl J Med*, 303:497–499, 1980.

the test performs well. But at lower prevalences, the positive predictive value drops to nearly zero, and the test is virtually useless for diagnosing disease.

Example—The predictive value of prostatic acid phosphatase for carcinoma of the prostate was studied using several different prevalences, corresponding to various clinical situations (Table 3.2). In the general population, where the prevalence of prostatic carcinoma is estimated to be 35/100,000, only 0.4% of men with positive test results actually have cancer. In high risk men (over 75 years old, where it is estimated that 500/100,000 would have cancer), 5.6% of positive tests represent cancer. In other words, if prostatic acid phosphatase were used as a screening test, even for these high risk men, 18 men with positive tests would have to be evaluated with additional tests in order to find one with cancer. However, when there is a strong clinical suspicion of malignancy because a nodule is felt, half of such men have prostatic cancer. In this situation, 93% of men with a positive test will have prostatic cancer (4).

Current efforts to prevent transmission of acquired immunodeficiency syndrome (AIDS) through blood products is another example of the effect of disease prevalence on positive predictive value.

Example—A blood test for antibodies to human immunodeficiency virus (HIV) is used to screen blood donors. At one cut-off point, the sensitivity is 97.75% and the specificity is 90.4%. In 1985, Barry et al. calculated the positive predictive value of the test by estimating that the prevalence of infectious units was no more than 1/10,000, and they showed that there would be 9250 false positive test results for every true positive result (5). Almost a thousand units would have to be screened to prevent one case of AIDS. The authors concluded that, for this emotionally charged subject, "careful adherence to the principles of diagnostic test evaluation will avoid unrealistic expectations."

But the situation is changing. As the prevalence of HIV infection increases in the general population, the positive predictive value of the screening test improves. In a publication a year later, the prevalence of infected units among 67,190 tested was 25/10,000, and at similar levels of sensitivity and specificity, the positive predictive value would be 2.5%, much higher than a few years before (6).

Estimating Prevalence

How can clinicians estimate the prevalence of disease among the patients in their setting in order to determine the predictive value of a test result? There are several sources of information: the medical literature, local data bases, and clinical judgment. Although the resulting estimate of prevalence is seldom very precise, error is not likely to be so great as to change clinical judgments that are based on the estimate. In any case, the process is bound to be more accurate than implicit judgment alone.

In general, prevalence is more important than sensitivity/specificity in determining predictive value. One reason why this is so is that prevalence commonly varies over a wider range. By current standards, clinicians are not particularly interested in tests with sensitivities and specificities much below 50%, but if both sensitivity and specificity are 99%, the test is considered a great one. In other words, in practical terms sensitivity and specificity rarely vary more than twofold. Prevalence of disease, however, can vary over a thousand-fold in various clinical settings. In Table 3.2, the prevalence of prostatic cancer varied from 35/100,000 to 50,000/100,000.

Increasing the Prevalence of Disease

Considering the relationship between the predictive value of a test and prevalence, it is obviously to the physician's advantage to apply diagnostic tests to patients with an increased likelihood of having the disease being sought. In fact as Figure 3.8 shows, diagnostic tests are most helpful when the presence of disease is neither very likely nor very unlikely. There are a variety of ways in which the probability of a disease can be increased before using a diagnostic test.

- **Referral process**

The referral process is one of the most common ways in which the probability of disease is increased. Teaching hospital wards, clinics, and emergency departments are frequently involved in this referral process, both because outside physicians formally refer patients and because patients informally refer themselves. The process increases the chance that significant disease will underlie patients' complaints. Therefore, relatively more aggressive use of diagnostic tests might be justified in these settings. In primary care practice, on the other hand, or among patients without complaints, the chance of finding disease is considerably smaller, and tests should be used more sparingly.

Example—While practicing in a military clinic, one of the authors saw hundreds of people with headache, rarely ordered diagnostic tests, and never encountered a patient with a severe underlying cause of headache. (It is unlikely that important conditions were missed because the clinic was virtually the only source of medical care for these patients and prolonged follow-up was available.) However, during the first week back in a medical residency, a patient visiting the hospital's emergency department because of a headache similar to the ones managed in the military was found to have a cerebellar abscess!

Because clinicians may work at different extremes of the prevalence spectrum at various times in their clinical practices, they should bear in mind that the intensity of diagnostic evaluation may need to be adjusted to suit the specific situation.

- **Selected demographic groups**

In a given setting, physicians can increase the yield of diagnostic tests by applying them to selected demographic groups known to be at higher risk for a disease. A man of 65 is 15 times more likely to have coronary artery disease as the cause of atypical chest pain than a woman of 30; thus, a particular diagnostic test for coronary disease, the electrocardiographic stress test, is less useful in confirming the diagnosis in the younger woman than in the older man (7). Similarly, a sickle test would obviously have a higher positive predictive value among blacks than among whites.

- **Specifics of the clinical situation**

The specifics of the clinical situation are clearly the strongest influence on the decision to order tests. Symptoms, signs, or even vague "clinical impressions" all raise or lower the probability of finding a disease. For example, a woman with pleurisy is more likely to have had a pulmonary embolus if she has tenderness and swelling in her leg and if she is on oral contraceptives than if she has none of these features. As a result, an abnormal lung scan is more likely to represent a pulmonary embolus in such a woman than in persons with pleurisy, but without any particular reason for having an embolus.

The value of applying specific diagnostic tests to persons more likely to have a particular illness is intuitively obvious to most doctors. Nevertheless, with the increasing availability of diagnostic tests, it is easy to adopt a less selective approach when ordering tests. However, the less selective the approach, the lower the prevalence of the disease is likely to be and the lower will be the positive predictive value of the test.

The magnitude of this effect can be larger than most of us might think.

Example—Factors that influence the interpretation of an abnormal electrocardiographic stress test are illustrated in Figure 3.9. It shows that the positive predictive value for coronary artery disease associated with an abnormal test can vary from 1.7 to 99.8%, depending on age, symptoms, and the degree of abnormality of the test. Thus, an exercise test in an asymptomatic 35-year-old man showing 1 mm ST segment depression will be a false positive test in over 98% of cases. The same test result in a 60-year-old man with typical angina by history will be associated with coronary artery disease in over 90% of cases (7).

Because of this effect, physicians must interpret similar test results differently in different clinical situations. In the previous example, a stress test in an asymptomatic 35-year-old man may be appropriate to confirm the absence of coronary artery disease, but usually will be misleading if it is used to search for unsuspected disease, as has been done among joggers, airline pilots, and business executives. The opposite applies to the 65-year-old man with typical angina. In this case, the test may be helpful in confirming disease but not in excluding disease. The test is most useful in intermediate situations, in which prevalence is neither very high nor very low. For example, a 60-year-old man with atypical chest pain has a 67% chance of coronary artery disease before stress testing (Fig. 3.9); but afterward, with greater than 2.5 mm ST segment depression, he has a 99% probability of coronary disease.

Because prevalence of disease is such a powerful determinant of how useful a diagnostic test for disease will be, clinicians must consider the probability of disease before ordering a test. The major means of doing so is by accurately interpreting the clinical context through careful observation during the history and physical examination. In an age when laboratory technology offers promise for solving complex diagnostic problems, we must still depend on medicine's oldest process—astute clinical observation.

Implications for the Medical Literature

Published descriptions of diagnostic tests often include, in addition to sensitivity and specificity, some conclusions about the interpretation of a positive or negative test—that is, predictive value. This is done, quite rightly, in order to provide information directly useful to clinicians. But the data for these publications are often gathered in university teaching hospitals where the prevalence of serious disease is relatively high. As a

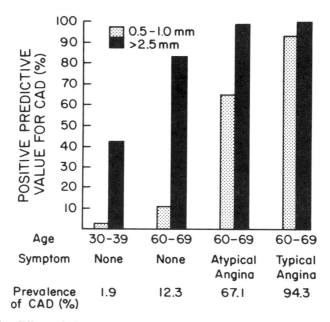

Figure 3.9. Effect of disease prevalence on positive predictive value of a diagnostic test. Probability of coronary artery disease in men according to age, symptoms, and depression of ST segment on electrocardiogram. (Data from Diamond GA, Forrester JS: Analysis of probability as an aid in the clinical diagnosis of coronary artery disease. *N Engl J Med* 300:1350–1358, 1979.

result, statements about predictive value in the medical literature may be misleading when the test is applied in less highly selected settings. What is worse, authors often compare the performance of a test in a number of patients known to have the disease and an equal number of patients without the disease. This is an efficient way to describe sensitivity and specificity. However, any reported positive predictive value from such studies may be falsely elevated because it has been determined for a group of patients in which the prevalence of disease is about 50%. Such a prevalence rarely corresponds to that found in naturally occurring groups of patients to which the test might be applied in practice (although such high prevalences can occur, as illustrated in Table 3.2).

LIKELIHOOD RATIOS

Likelihood ratios are an alternative way of describing the performance of a diagnostic test. They summarize the same kind of information as sensitivity/specificity and can be used to calculate the probability of disease after a positive or negative test.

Odds

Because use of likelihood ratios depend on odds, to understand them it is first necessary to distinguish odds from probability. *Probability*—used to express sensitivity, specificity, and predictive value—is the proportion of people in whom a particular characteristic, such as a positive test, is present. *Odds*, on the other hand, is the ratio of two probabilities. Odds and probability contain the same information, but express it differently. The two can be interconverted using simple formulae:

$$\text{Odds} = \frac{\text{probability of event}}{1 - \text{probability of event}} \quad \text{Probability} = \frac{\text{odds}}{1 + \text{odds}}$$

These terms should be familiar to most readers because they are used in everyday conversation. For example, we may say that the odds are 4:1 that the University of North Carolina "Tar Heels" basketball team will win tonight or that they have an 80% probability of winning.

Definitions

The *likelihood ratio* for a particular value of a diagnostic test is defined as the probability of that test result in the presence of disease divided by the probability of the result in people without disease. Likelihood ratios express how many times more (or less) likely a test result is to be found in diseased, as compared to nondiseased, people. If a test is dichotomous (positive/negative) two types of likelihood ratios describe its ability to discriminate between diseased and nondiseased people; one is associated with a positive test and the other with a negative test (Figs. 3.2 and 3.10).

In the pharyngitis example (Fig. 3.3), the data can be used to calculate likelihood ratios for streptococcal pharyngitis in the presence of a positive or negative test (clinical diagnosis). A positive test is about 2½ times more likely to be made in the presence of streptococcal pharyngitis than in the absence of it. If the clinicians believed streptococcal pharyngitis was not present, the likelihood ratio for this negative test was .39; the odds were about 1:2.6 that a negative clinical diagnosis would be made in the presence of streptococcal pharyngitis as compared to the absence of it.

Uses of Likelihood Ratios

Pretest probability (prevalence) can be converted to pretest odds using the formula presented above. Likelihood ratio can then be used to convert pretest odds to posttest odds, by means of the following formula:

Pretest Odds × Likelihood Ratio = Posttest Odds

Posttest odds can in turn be converted back to a probability, again using the formula described under the section on "Odds." In these relationships, pretest odds contains the same information as prior probability (prevalence), likelihood ratios the same as sensitivity/specificity, and posttest odds the same as positive predictive value (posttest probability).

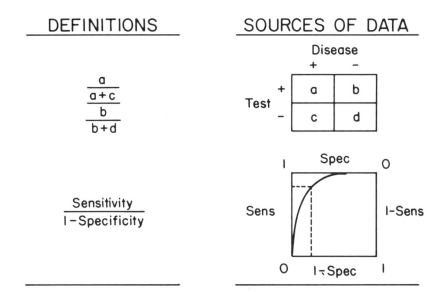

DEFINITIONS

SOURCES OF DATA

Figure 3.10. Likelihood ratios for positive tests: definitions and sources of data.

The main advantage of likelihood ratios is that they make it easier for us to go beyond the simple and clumsy classification of a test result as either abnormal or normal, as is usually done when describing the accuracy of a diagnostic test only in terms of sensitivity and specificity at a single cut-off point. Obviously, disease is more likely in the presence of an extremely abnormal test result than it is for a marginal one. With likelihood ratios, it is possible to summarize the information contained in a test result at different levels. One can define likelihood ratios for any number of test results, over the entire range of possible values. In this way, information represented by the degree of abnormality, rather than the crude presence or absence of it, is not discarded. Thus, likelihood ratios can accommodate the common and reasonable clinical practice of putting more weight on extremely high (or low) test results than on borderline ones, when estimating the probability (or odds) that a particular disease is present.

Example—How accurate is serum thyroxine (T_4) alone as a test for hypothyroidism? Goldstein and Mushlin addressed this question in a study of 120 ambulatory general medical patients suspected of having hypothyroidism. Patients were diagnosed as being hypothyroid if serum thyrotropin (TSH) was elevated, and subsequent evaluations, including other thyroid tests and response to treatment, were consistent with hypothyroidism. The authors studied the initial T_4 level in 27 patients with hypothyroidism and 93 patients who were found not to have it to determine how accurately the simple test alone might have diagnosed hypothyroidism.

As expected, likelihood ratios for hypothyroidism were highest for low levels of T_4 and lowest for high levels (Table 3.3). The lowest values in the distribution of

Table 3.3
Distribution of Values for Serum Thyroxine in Hypothyroid and Normal Patients, with Calculation of Likelihood Ratios[a]

TOTAL SERUM THYROXINE	PATIENTS WITH TEST RESULT		LIKELIHOOD RATIO
	HYPOTHYROID	NORMAL	
μg/dl	no. (%)	no. (%)	
<1.1	2 (7.4)		↑
1.1–2.0	3 (11.1)		RULED IN
2.1–3.0	1 (3.7)		
3.1–4.0	8 (29.6)		↓
4.1–5.0	4 (14.8)	1 (1.1)	13.8
5.1–6.0	4 (14.8)	6 (6.5)	2.3
6.1–7.0	3 (11.1)	11 (11.8)	.9
7.1–8.0	2 (7.4)	19 (20.4)	.4
8.1–9.0		17 (18.3)	↑
9.1–10.		20 (21.5)	
10.1–11		11 (11.8)	RULED OUT
11.1–12		4 (4.3)	
>12		4 (4.3)	
Total	27 (100)	93 (100)	↓

[a] From Goldstein BJ, Mushlin AI: Use of a single thyroxine test to evaluate ambulatory medical patients for suspected hypothyroidism. *J Gen Intern Med* 2: 20–24, 1987.

T_4s (<4.0 μg/dl) were not seen in patients without hypothyroidism—that is, these levels ruled in the diagnosis. The highest levels (>8.0 μg/dl) were not seen in patients with hypothyroidism—that is, the presence of these levels ruled out the disease.

The authors concluded that "it may be possible to achieve cost savings without loss of diagnostic accuracy by using a single total T_4 measurement for the initial evaluation of suspected hypothyroidism in selected patients (8).

A set of likelihood ratios contains all the information in an ROC curve for the same test. Indeed, likelihood ratios at any given cut-off point can be obtained from an ROC curve (Fig. 3.10).

Likelihood ratios have several other advantages over sensitivity/specificity as a description of test performance. The information contributed by the test is summarized in one number instead of two. The calculations necessary for obtaining posttest odds from pretest odds are easy. Also, likelihood ratios are particularly well suited for describing the overall probability of disease when a series of diagnostic tests is used (see below).

Likelihood ratios also have disadvantages. One must use odds, not probabilities, and most of us find thinking in terms of odds more difficult than probabilities. Also, the conversion from probability to odds and back requires math or the use of a nomogram, which partly offsets the simplicity of calculating the LRs themselves.

MULTIPLE TESTS

Because clinicians commonly use imperfect diagnostic tests, with less than 100% sensitivity and specificity and intermediate likelihood ratios, a single test frequently results in a probability of disease that is neither very high nor very low—for example, somewhere between 10% and 90%. Usually it is not acceptable to stop the diagnostic process at such a point. Would a physician or patient be satisfied with the conclusion that the patient has a 50/50 chance of having carcinoma of the colon? Or that an asymptomatic 35-year-old man with 2.5 mm ST segment depression on a stress test has a 42% chance of coronary artery disease (Fig. 3.9)? Even for less deadly diseases, such as hypothyroidism, tests with intermediate post-test probability are of little help. The physician is ordinarily bound to raise or lower the probability of disease substantially in such situations—unless, of course, the diagnostic possibilities are all trivial, nothing could be done about the result, or the risk of proceeding further is prohibitive. When these exceptions do not apply, the doctor will want to proceed with further tests.

When multiple tests are performed and all are positive or all are negative, the interpretation is straightforward. All too often, however, some are positive and others are negative. Interpretation is then more complicated. This section will discuss the principles by which multiple tests are interpreted.

Multiple tests can be applied in two general ways (Fig. 3.11). They can

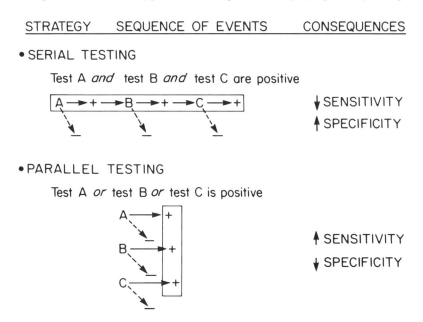

Figure 3.11. Serial and parallel testing.

be used in *parallel* (i.e., all at once) and a positive result of any test considered evidence for disease. Or they can be done *serially* (i.e., consecutively) each based on the results of the previous test. For serial testing, all tests must give a positive result for the diagnosis to be made, because the diagnostic process is stopped when a negative result is obtained.

Parallel Tests

Physicians usually order tests in parallel when rapid assessment is necessary, as in hospitalized or emergency patients, or for ambulatory patients who cannot return easily because they have come from a long distance for evaluation.

Multiple tests in parallel increase the sensitivity, and therefore the negative predictive value, for a given disease prevalence above those of each individual test. On the other hand, specificity and positive predictive value are lowered. That is, disease is less likely to be missed (parallel testing is probably one reason referral centers seem to diagnose disease that local physicians miss), but false positive diagnoses are also more likely to be made (thus, the propensity for overdiagnosing in such centers as well). These relationships are demonstrated in Table 3.4.

Parallel testing is particularly useful when the clinician is faced with the need for a very sensitive test, but has available only two or more relatively insensitive ones. By using the tests in parallel, the net effect is a more sensitive diagnostic strategy. The price, however, is evaluation or treatment of some patients without the disease.

Example—Diagnosis of deep vein thrombosis in the leg remains a difficult clinical challenge. The most accurate test (i.e., gold standard) is venography involving injection of radiographic dye into the venous system of the leg. But venography is both expensive and somewhat risky; many physicians are reluctant to use it in every patient suspected of having deep vein thrombophlebitis.

As an alternative approach, two less accurate tests were used in parallel: impedance plethysmography and leg scanning after an injection of ^{125}I fibrinogen.

Table 3.4
Effect of Parallel and Serial Testing on Sensitivity, Specificity, and Predictive Value of Test Combinations

TEST	SENSITIVITY	SPECIFICITY	POSITIVE PREDICTIVE VALUE[a]	NEGATIVE PREDICTIVE VALUE[a]
	%	%	%	%
A	80	60	33	92
B	90	90	69	97
A or B (Parallel)	98	54	35	99
A and B (Serial)	72	96	82	93

[a] For 20% prevalence.

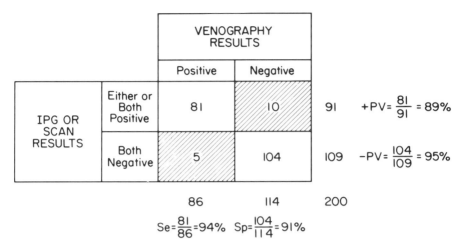

Figure 3.12. Example of parallel testing for the diagnosis of deep vein thrombosis. Two tests, leg scanning and impedance plethysmography, are used and the results compared to venography, the gold standard. Sensitivity of the combination is 94%. (Data from Hull R, Hirsh J, Sackett DL, Powers P, Turpie AGG, Walker I: Combined use of leg scanning and impedance plethysmography in suspected venous thrombosis. An alternative to venography. *N Engl J Med* 296:1497–1500, 1977.)

Although neither test alone was as sensitive and specific as venography, using the two together achieved a sensitivity of 94% and a specificity of 91% (Fig. 3.12).

In this situation, a parallel testing strategy could improve patient care by providing an accurate, safe, and less expensive alternative to venography (9).

Serial Testing

Physicians most commonly use serial testing strategies in clinical situations where rapid assessment of patients is not required, such as in office practices and hospital clinics in which ambulatory patients are followed over time. Serial testing is also used when some of the tests are expensive or risky, these tests being employed only after simpler and safer tests suggest the presence of disease. Serial testing leads to less laboratory utilization than parallel testing because additional evaluation is contingent on prior test results. However, serial testing takes more time because additional tests are ordered as the results of previous ones become available.

Serial testing maximizes specificity and positive predictive value, but lowers sensitivity and the negative predictive value. One ends up surer that positive test results represent disease, but runs an increased risk that disease will be missed. Serial testing is particularly useful when none of the individual tests available to a clinician is highly specific.

If a physician is going to use two tests in series, everything else being

Table 3.5
Effect of Sequence in Serial Testing: A Then B versus B Then A[a]

Prevalence of Disease

Number of patients tested	1000
Number of patients with disease	200 (20% prevalence)

Sensitivity and Specificity of Tests

Test	Sensitivity	Specificity
A	80	90
B	90	80

Sequence of Testing

Begin with Test A

		Disease +	Disease −	
A	+	160	80	240
	−	40	720	760
		200	800	1000

240 Patients Retested with B

		Disease +	Disease −	
B	+	144	16	160
	−	16	64	80
		160	80	240

Begin with Test B

		Disease +	Disease −	
B	+	180	160	340
	−	20	640	660
		200	800	1000

340 Patients Retested with A

		Disease +	Disease −	
A	+	144	16	160
	−	46	144	180
		180	160	340

[a] Note that in both sequences the same number of patients are identified as diseased (160), and the same number of true positives (144) are identified. But when Test A (with the higher specificity) is used first, fewer patients are retested. The lower sensitivity of Test A does not adversely affect the final result.

equal, the test with the highest specificity should be used first. Table 3.5 shows the effect of sequence on serial testing. Test A is more specific than test B, whereas B is more sensitive than A. By using A first, fewer patients are subjected to both tests, even though equal numbers of diseased patients are diagnosed, regardless of the sequence of tests.

Assumption of Independence

When multiple tests are used, it is often assumed that the additional information contributed by each test is independent of that already available from the preceding ones—that is, the next test does not simply duplicate known information. In fact, this assumption underlies the entire approach to predictive value we have discussed. The assumption is likely to be correct when a manifestation of disease changes with time, as when stool is tested for occult blood repeatedly on the belief that an occult malignancy bleeds intermittently. Independence of tests also is likely if the tests are measuring different phenomena. In the example of plethysmography and leg scanning for diagnosing deep vein thrombophlebitis, there is evidence that plethysmography detects thromboses in the thigh, whereas leg scanning is better at finding thromboses in the calf. Thus, these tests may complement each other.

However, it seems unlikely that multiple tests for most diseases are truly independent of one another. If the assumption that the tests are completely independent is wrong, calculation of the probability of disease from several tests would tend to overestimate the tests' value.

Serial Likelihood Ratios

When a series of tests is used, an overall probability can be calculated, using the likelihood ratio for each test result, as shown in Figure 3.13. The prevalence of disease before testing is first converted to pretest odds. As each test is done, the posttest odds of one becomes the pretest odds for the next. In the end, a new probability of disease is found that takes into account the information contributed by all the tests in the series.

CLINICAL DECISION MAKING

Clinical decision making requires weighing the benefits and costs of an action. Both the benefits and costs should be broadly defined to include all of the important consequences of the decision. *Benefits* are the outcomes we have been discussing so far in this book—in general, to relieve suffering, restore function, and prevent untimely death. *Costs* often refer to money, but also include side effects, reduction in length of life, and loss of other resources, e.g., time, energy, good will.

Often it is necessary to make a trade-off among the various benefits and costs of an action—for example, the length versus quality of life on chemotherapy or short-term risk versus potential for long-term gains with surgery. This trade-off has traditionally been done without formal groundrules or much use of explicit probabilities. It is called "clinical judgment" and is what we learn at the bedside and in the clinics. If our teachers are good, so are the results.

In recent years, methods for quantitative decision making have been introduced into medicine. The most commonly used strategies are decision analysis, cost effectiveness analysis, and cost benefit analysis. These meth-

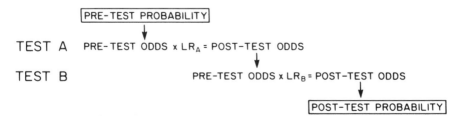

Figure 3.13. Use of likelihood ratios in series.

ods first explicitly define the important factors in a decision and then its consequences, assign probabilities to events and numbers to value judgments, such as quality of life, and finally proceed by formal, logical rules to derive the best course of action. Quantitative decision making has been used to define the most effective and efficient way to deal with specific problems in individual patients (*clinical policy*) or for allocating resources to larger groups of people, such as communities or political jurisdictions (*public policy*).

We indicated in Chapter 1 that the main purpose of this book was to consider the groundrules that determine the quality of information on which clinical decisions (involving both value judgments and data) can be based. There are excellent books about clinical decision making itself (see Suggested Readings) and the related topic, medical economics. Here, we will simply outline the main features of three approaches to quantitative decision making.

Decision Analysis

In *decision analysis*, one sets, out alternative courses of action and then calculates which choice is likely to result in the most valued outcome, based on estimates of probability for each branch in the sequences of events and judgments about the relative value of the possible outcomes. The basic steps are clearly presented elsewhere (10) and are only described briefly below.

1. *Create a decision tree.* Clinical decision analysis begins with a patient who poses a dilemma. Which of the possible courses of action should be taken? The tree starts with these alternative decisions, then branches out to include all of the important consequences of those decisions, and ends with the clinically important outcomes. Branch points involve either patient care decisions ("choice nodes," indicated by squares) or spontaneous events ("chance nodes," indicated by circles). Although there are an infinite number of sequences of events and outcomes, usually only a small number are truly important and are reasonably likely to occur. To make the analysis manageable, it is necessary to "prune" the tree so that only the most important branches are included—typically no more than several branch points.
2. *Assign probabilities to chance nodes.* These probabilities can be estimated by referring to the medical literature, local experience (e.g., a local data bank), or the opinion of experts. The probabilities may be imprecise, but no more so than without decision analysis.
3. *Assign utilities to the outcomes.* The units are arbitrary, but must be on an interval scale—for example, 0–100. One way to do this is to rank the outcomes in order of their value and then decide on the size of the difference between them. In most situations, the point of reference should be the patient's preferences, just as it is for any clinical decision. It may seem awkward to put a number on the respective values of the various outcomes—death, suffering, loss of function—especially when

they are measured in different units, such as the length and quality of life. But we do attach values to outcomes in any case, and the numbers only make the values explicit.

4. *Calculate the expected utilities* for the alternative courses of action. Starting with utilities (at the end of the branches, to the right), multiply utilities by probabilities for each branch and add branches at each node in succession until the expected utility at the main branch point, the decision that has to be made, is reached.

5. *Select the choice* with the highest expected utility.

6. *Sensitivity analysis.* Estimates of probabilities and utilities were uncertain in the first place. The final step in decision analysis is to see how the results of the analysis change as these estimates are varied over a range of plausible values. That is, one must find out how "sensitive" the decision is to imprecision in the estimates. Sensitivity analysis indicates which points in the sequence of events have the most effect on the decision and how large the effect might be.

Example—Weinstein et al. (11) analysed the decisions necessary to manage a 68-year-old man who has a long history of peripheral vascular disease. After a penetrating foot injury he develops an infection and possibly gangrene. Should his clinicians recommend immediate amputation below the knee or delay surgery, treat medically, and hope that an amputation can be avoided altogether—at the risk that a worse outcome, above the knee amputation or even death from sepsis, might result? Figure 3.14 shows the decision tree that the authors use to analyse the options. You can improve your understanding of decision analysis by working through the six steps described above while referring to this specific tree.

Advocates of decision analysis point out that it has several advantages over the usual way of making clinical decisions. It forces the decision

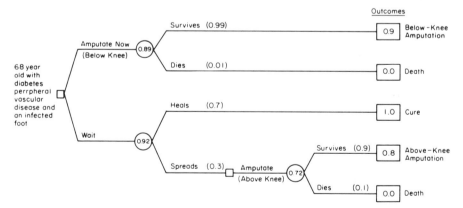

Figure 3.14. Example of a decision tree. Management of a 68-year-old man with diabetes, peripheral vascular disease, and an infected foot. (Data from Weinstein MC, Fineberg HV, et al: *Clinical Decision Analysis.* Philadelphia, WB Saunders Co, 1980.)

maker to define explicitly alternative courses of action, their potential consequences, and the values attached to outcomes of care. Probabilities are stated outright, rather than implied (imprecisely), as is usually the case. Also, the process is logical, and that appeals to the intellect.

Detractors note that decision analysis takes time—usually hours per case—and there is rarely enough time in a busy clinician's life. Pruning the tree may remove important branches. Also, does decision analysis really obtain better results than conventional decision making? The method has rarely been put to this test. After all, it is no more acceptable to justify decision analysis by the elegance of the process than it is to say that one can predict the course of disease or the results of treatment from a knowledge of pathophysiology alone.

Cost-Effectiveness Analysis

As the name implies, *cost-effectiveness analysis* is a way of deciding on the relative merits of alternative courses of action by comparing what they cost (in money) to achieve a given health effect. Alternatively, one can compare the outcomes achieved for a given cost.

Costs are characterized in terms of a single, common unit—money. Usually a broad view is taken, including all the costs—direct and indirect—that might reasonably be incurred by a course of action. This might include the costs of clinicians' services, hospital room, laboratory and radiologic tests, medications, side effects, travel to obtain medical care, lost wages, and the like. If morbidity and mortality are taken into account, and they should be, they must be converted to their monetary value. This is, of course, less satisfying. Note that charges, the amount patients (or others on their behalf) are billed for a particular service, are not the same as costs; charges may be substantially more or less than actual costs, because of the way the books happen to be kept.

Effectiveness is expressed as a health outcome—for example, year of life saved, disease prevented or cured, function restored, etc.

Example—How should serious infection be treated when the responsible organism has not been isolated? Modern, single-dose, broad spectrum antibiotics, such as third-generation cephalosporins, cost more to purchase, but are less toxic than conventional, multidrug regimens and may be nearly as effective. Weinstein et al. studied the costs and effectiveness of treatment choices for three serious classes of infection: hospital-acquired pneumonia, intra-abdominal infection, and sepsis of unknown origin. They took a broad view of costs, including acquisition of the drug, preparation, administration, monitoring, and toxicity. Effectiveness was estimated by a panel of experts.

In general, the total cost of using third-generation cephalosporins was similar or less than other regimens. Estimates of effectiveness (loss of life expectancy) for the regimens differed for the various regimens but not in a large way. Effects of toxicity on length of life were small compared with possible differences in the loss of life from infection if drug regimens differed in efficacy. Cost effectiveness was sensitive to assumptions about effectiveness that presently, in the absence of many studies of the new agents, is relatively uncertain.

This analysis suggests that differences among the regimens is not great, considering the current state of knowledge, and illustrates the value of taking a comprehensive view of costs for alternative courses of action (12).

Cost-Benefit Analysis

In *cost-benefit analysis*, both costs and benefits of alternative courses of action are expressed in the same units of value, money. The output is cost:benefit ratios, net benefits, or net costs.

Cost-benefit analyses have been most useful for guiding policy decisions—for example, whether vaccination programs for pneumococcus or pertussis result in net savings to society. These analyses are less often found in the clinical literature, perhaps because it is particularly difficult to describe the accomplishments of health care purely in terms of money gained or lost.

SUMMARY

Diagnostic test performance is judged by comparing the results of the test to the presence of disease in a two-by-two table. All four cells of the table must be filled. When estimating the sensitivity and specificity of a new diagnostic test from information in the medical literature, there must be a "gold standard" to which the accuracy of the test is compared. The diseased and nondiseased subjects should both resemble the kinds of patients for whom the test might be useful in practice. In addition, knowledge of the final diagnosis should not bias the interpretation of the test results or vice versa. Likelihood ratios are another way of describing the accuracy of a diagnostic test. Changing the cut-off point between normal and abnormal changes sensitivity and specificity.

The predictive value of a test is the most relevant characteristic when clinicians interpret test results. It is determined not only by sensitivity and specificity of the test but also by the prevalence of the disease, which may change from setting to setting.

Usually it is necessary to use several tests, either in parallel or in series, to achieve acceptable diagnostic certainty. Clinical decision making can be guided by quantitative methods: decision analysis, cost-effectiveness analysis, and cost-benefit analysis.

REFERENCES

1. Butler RL: *Wood for Wood-Carvers and Craftsmen.* New York, AS Barnes and Co, 1974.
2. Bartrum RJ Jr, Crow HC, Foote SR: Ultrasonic and radiographic cholecystography. *N Engl J Med* 296:538–541, 1977.
3. Cooperberg PL, Burhenne HJ: Real-time ultrasonography: diagnostic technique of choice in calculous gallbladder disease. *N Engl J Med* 302:1277–1279, 1980.

4. Watson RA, Tang DB: The predictive value of prostatic acid phosphatase as a screening test for prostatic cancer. *N Engl J Med* 303:497–499, 1980.

5. Barry MJ, Mulley AG, Singer DE: Screening for HTLV III antibodies: the relation between prevalence and positive predictive value and its social consequences. *JAMA* 253:3395, 1985.

6. Ward JW, Grindon AJ, Feorino PM, Schable C, Parvin M, Allen JR: Laboratory and epidemiologic evaluation of an enzyme immunoassay for antibodies to HTLV 111. *JAMA* 256:357–61, 1986.

7. Diamond GA, Forrester JS: Analysis of probability as an aid in the clinical diagnosis of coronary artery disease. *N Engl J Med* 300:1350–1358, 1979.

8. Goldstein BJ, Mushlin AI: Use of a single thyroxine test to evaluate ambulatory medical patients for suspected hypothyroidism. *J Gen Intern Med* 2:20–24, 1987.

9. Hull R, Hirsh J, Sackett DL, Powers P, Turpie AGG, Walker I: Combined use of leg scanning and impedance plethysmography in suspected venous thrombosis. An alternative to venography. *N Engl J Med* 296:1497–1500, 1977.

10. Sackett DL, Haynes RB, Tugwell P: *Clinical Epidemiology. A Basic Science for Clinical Medicine.* Boston, Little, Brown and Co, 1985.

11. Weinstein MC, Fineberg HV, Elstein AS, Frazier HS, Neuhauser D, Neutra RR, McNeil BJ: *Clinical Decision Analysis.* Philadelphia, WB Saunders Co, 1980.

12. Weinstein MC, Read JL, MacKay DN, Kresel JJ, Ashley H, Halvorsen KT, Hutchings HC: Cost-effective choice of antimicrobial therapy for serious infection. *J Gen Intern Med* 1:351–363, 1986.

SUGGESTED READINGS

Cebul RD, Beck LH: *Teaching Clinical Decision Making.* New York, Praeger, 1985.

Department of Clinical Epidemiology and Biostatistics, McMaster University: Interpretation of diagnostic data. V. How to do it with simple math. *Can Med Assoc J* 129:22–29, 1983. (Also in Sackett DL, Haynes RB, Tugwell P: *Clinical Epidemiology. A Basic Science for Clinical Medicine.* Boston, Little, Brown and Co, 1985.)

Fagan TJ: Nomogram for Bayes' theorem (letter). *N Engl J Med* 293:257, 1975.

Fletcher RH: Carcinoembryonic antigen. *Ann Intern Med* 104:66–73, 1986.

Griner PF, Mayewski RJ, Mushlin AI, Greenland P: Selection and interpretation of diagnostic tests and procedures. Principles and applications. *Ann Intern Med* 94: 453–600, 1981.

Griner PF, Panzer RJ, Greenland P: *Clinical Diagnosis and the Laboratory: Logical Strategies for Common Medical Problems.* Chicago. Year Book, 1986.

McNeil BJ, Abrams HL (eds): *Brigham and Women's Hospital Handbook of Diagnostic Imaging.* Boston, Little, Brown and Co, 1986.

Pauker SG, Kassirer JP: Clinical application of decision analysis: a detailed illustration. *Semin Nucl Med* 8:324–335, 1978.

Sheps SB, Schechter MT: The assessment of diagnostic tests. A survey of current medical research. *JAMA* 252:2418–2422, 1984.

Sox HC Jr: Probability theory in the use of diagnostic tests. An introduction to critical study of the literature. *Ann Intern Med* 104:60–66, 1986.

Sox HC, Jr., Blatt M, Higgins MC, Marton KI: *Medical Decision Making.* London, Butterworths, 1987.

Wasson JH, Sox HC Jr, Neff RK, Goldman L: Clinical prediction rules. Applications and methodological standards. *N Engl J Med* 313:793–799, 1985.

Weinstein MC, Fineberg HV, Elstein AS, Frazier HS, Neuhauser D, Neutra RR, McNeil BJ: *Clinical Decision Analysis.* Philadelphia, WB Saunders, 1980.

APPENDIX 3.1. MAIN QUESTIONS FOR DETERMINING THE VALIDITY OF STUDIES OF DIAGNOSTIC TESTS[a]

1. Is the *test procedure:*
   a. Fully *described?*
   b. *Unbiased* (Not affected by knowledge of the presence or absence of disease)?
2. Is the true presence or absence of disease (*"gold standard"*) established for all patients, i.e., both for those with and without an abnormal test result?
3. Is a statistic for test accuracy reported?
   a. *Sensitivity/specificity or likelihood ratio* (LR)
   b. For tests with a range of potential values, is the change in accuracy when *moving the cut-point* between normal and abnormal described? (expressed as ROC curve or multiple LRs)
4. Is there a description of the *spectrum of diseased and nondiseased patients* used to establish test accuracy, including effect of:
   a. Stage and severity of disease?
   b. Presenting symptoms and diseases among "nondiseased" group? (To be clinically useful, accuracy should be established for patients with presenting symptoms similar to those with the disease in question.)
5. *Is there a description of predictive value* at various prevalences of disease, particularly those in which the test is ordinarily used? (Note: this information is not essential; the reader can estimate prevalence and calculate predictive value if the other information is present.)

---

[a] These questions are not meant to be all-inclusive, nor to replace independent, critical thinking. They are a rough guideline, including only the most basic elements of a sound study.

chapter 4

FREQUENCY

In Chapter 1, we outlined the central questions facing clinicians as they care for patients. In this chapter, we will build a foundation for the evidence that clinicians use to guide their diagnostic and therapeutic decisions. Let us introduce the subject with a patient.

A 22-year-old man presents with sore throat, fever, and malaise of 2 days duration. Further history indicates no exposure to sick persons and no prior history of significant illness. Physical examination reveals a temperature of 38°C, an erythematous pharynx with whitish exudate and tonsillar enlargement, tender anterior cervical lymph nodes, and no other positive findings.

In planning further diagnosis and treatment, the clinician must deal with several questions:

1. How likely is the patient to have streptococcal pharyngitis?
2. If the patient has streptococcal infection, how likely is he to develop a serious complication, such as acute rheumatic fever or acute glomerulonephritis?
3. How likely is penicillin treatment to prevent rheumatic fever or glomerulonephritis?
4. If the patient is treated with penicillin, how likely is an important allergic reaction?

Depending on the answers to these questions, the physician may treat with penicillin right away, obtain a throat culture and await the result, or offer only symptomatic treatment.

Each of these questions concerns the likelihood or commonness of a clinical event under certain circumstances. The questions could all be recast so as to ask—How frequently do streptococcal pharyngitis or rheumatic fever or penicillin allergic reactions occur under particular circumstances?

The evidence required to manage this patient rationally—the likelihood or frequency of disease or outcomes—is, in general, the kind of evidence needed to answer most clinical questions. Decisions are guided by the commonness of things. Usually, they depend on the relative commonness of things under alternative circumstances: in the presence of a positive test versus a negative test or after treatment A versus treatment B. Because the commonness of disease, improvement, deterioration, cure, or death forms the basis for answering most clinical questions, this chapter will examine measures of clinical frequency.

ASSIGNING NUMBERS TO PROBABILITY STATEMENTS

Physicians often communicate probabilities as words—"usually," "sometimes," "rarely," etc.—rather than as numbers. Substituting words for numbers is convenient and avoids making a precise statement when one is uncertain about a probability. However, it has been shown that there is little agreement about the meanings of commonly used words for frequency.

Example—Physicians were asked to estimate the likelihood of disease for each of 30 expressions of probability found by reviewing radiology and laboratory reports. There was great difference of opinion for each expression. Probabilities for "consistent with" ranged from .18 to .98; for "unlikely," the range was .01 to .93. These data support the authors' assertion that "difference of opinion among physicians regarding the management of a problem may reflect differences in the meaning ascribed to words used to define probability" (1).

Patients also assign widely varying values for expressions of probability. In another study, highly skilled and professional workers thought "usually" referred to probabilities of .35 to 1.0 (± 2 standard deviations from the mean); "rarely" meant to them a probability of 0 to .15 (2).

Thus, substituting words for numbers diminishes the information conveyed. We advocate using numbers whenever possible.

PREVALENCE AND INCIDENCE

In general, clinically relevant measures of the frequency of events are fractions in which the numerator is the number of patients experiencing the outcome (cases) and the denominator is the number of people in whom the outcome could have occurred. Such fractions are of course proportions, but by common usage, are often referred to as "rates." As ex-students of physics, we recognize the incorrectness of this use of rate, but there seems to be little chance that it will disappear.

Clinicians encounter two measures of commonness—prevalence and incidence.

A *prevalence* is the fraction (proportion) of a group possessing a clinical condition at a given point in time.[a] Prevalence is measured by surveying a

---

[a] There are two kinds of prevalence. *Point prevalence* is measured at a single point in time for each person, although not necessarily for all the people in the defined population. *Period prevalence* is a count of the proportion of cases that were present at any time during a period of time.

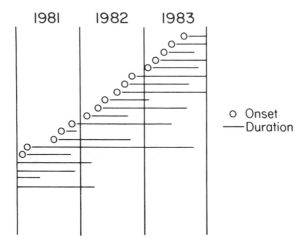

Figure 4.1. Occurrence of disease in 100 people at risk from 1981–1983.

defined population containing people with and without the condition of interest, at a single point in time.

An *incidence* is the fraction or proportion of a group initially free of the condition that develops it over a given period of time. As described later in this chapter and in greater detail in Chapter 5, incidence is measured by identifying a susceptible group of people (i.e., people free of the disease or the outcome) and examining them periodically over an interval of time so as to discover and count new cases that develop during the interval.

To illustrate the differences between prevalence and incidence, Figure 4.1 shows the occurrence of disease in a group of 100 people over the course of 3 years (1981, 1982, 1983). As time passes, individuals in the group develop the disease. They remain in this state until they either recover or die. In the 3 years, 16 people suffer the onset of disease and 4 already had it. Eighty do not develop disease and do not appear on the figure.

At the beginning of 1981 there are four cases, so the prevalence at that point in time is 4/100. If all 100 individuals, including prior cases, are examined at the beginning of each year, one can compute the prevalence at those points in time. At the beginning of 1982, the prevalence is 5/100 because two of the pre-1981 cases lingered on into 1982 and two of the new cases developing in 1981 terminated (hopefully in a cure) before the examination at the start of 1982. Prevalences can be computed for each of the other two annual examinations, and assuming that none of the original 100 people died, moved away, or refused examination, these prevalences are 7/100 at the beginning of 1983 and 5/100 at the beginning of 1984.

To calculate the incidence of new cases developing in the population, we consider only the 96 individuals free of the disease at the beginning of 1981 and what happens to them over the next 3 years. Five new cases developed in 1981; six new cases developed in 1982, and five additional new cases developed in 1983. The 3-year incidence of the disease is all new cases developing in the 3 years (16) divided by the number of susceptible individuals at the beginning of the follow-up period (96), or 16/96 in 3 years. What would be the annual incidences for 1981, 1982, and 1983, respectively? Remembering to remove the previous cases from the denominator, the annual incidences would be 5/96 for 1981, 6/91 for 1982, and 5/85 for 1983.

Every measure of disease frequency of necessity contains some indication of time. With measures of prevalence, time is assumed to be instantaneous, as in a single frame from a motion picture. Prevalence depicts the situation at that point in time for each patient even though it may, in reality, have taken several weeks or months to collect observations on the various people in the group studied. For incidence, time is the essence because it defines the interval during which susceptible subjects were monitored for the emergence of the event of interest. Two distinct approaches to the assessment of incidence are encountered in the medical literature and are described below.

Table 4.1 summarizes the characteristics of incidence and prevalence. Although the distinctions between the two seem clear, the literature is replete with misuses of the terms, particularly incidence (3).

Why is it important to know the difference between prevalence and incidence? Because they are answers to two different questions: (1) What proportion of a group of people have a condition? and (2) at what rate do new cases arise in a group of people as time passes? The answer to one question cannot be obtained directly from the answer to the other.

MEASURING PREVALENCE AND INCIDENCE

Prevalence Studies

The prevalence of disease is measured by surveying a group of people, some of whom are diseased at that point in time while others are healthy.

Table 4.1
Characteristics of Incidence and Prevalence

	Incidence	Prevalance
Numerator	New cases occurring during a period of time among a group initially free of disease	All cases counted on a single survey or examination of a group
Denominator	All susceptible people present at the beginning of the period	All people examined, including cases and noncases
Time	Duration of the period	Single point
How measured	Cohort study (see Chapter 5)	Prevalence (cross-sectional) study

The fraction or proportion of the group who are diseased (i.e., cases) constitutes the prevalence of the disease.

Such one-shot examinations or surveys of a population of individuals including cases and noncases are called *prevalence* studies. Another term is *cross-sectional studies* because people are studied at a point (cross-section) in time. They are among the more common types of research designs reported in the medical literature, constituting approximately one-third of original articles in major medical journals.

The following is an example of a typical prevalence study.

Example—What is the prevalence of rheumatoid arthritis in the general population? To answer this question, O'Sullivan and Cathcart surveyed all 4552 of the people over age 15 living in a small town in Massachusetts. Each participant completed a questionnaire and underwent an examination that included a medical history, physical examination, and blood tests. The presence of rheumatoid arthritis was defined by explicit criteria in general use: the New York and the American Rheumatology Association (ARA) criteria.

Of the 77% of the defined population who participated, the prevalence of rheumatoid arthritis was about 4 cases per 1000 by the New York criteria and 26 per 1000 by the ARA criteria (4).

Incidence Studies

In contrast to prevalence, incidence is measured by first identifying a population free of the event of interest and then following them through time with periodic examinations to determine occurrences of the event. This process, also called a cohort study, will be discussed in detail in Chapter 5.

Up until now, we have defined incidence as the rate of new events in a group of people of fixed size, all of whom are observed over a period of time. This is called *cumulative incidence* because new cases are accumulated over time.

Example—The death rate after acute respiratory failure complicating chronic respiratory disease was studied by observing the survival of 145 patients. After 1 year, 90 patients had died, for a death rate (incidence of death) of 90/145/year. After 5 years, the death rate was 122/145/5 years (5).

A second approach to incidence is to measure the number of new cases emerging in an ever-changing population, where people are under study and susceptible for varying lengths of time. Typical examples are clinical trials of chronic treatment in which eligible patients are enrolled over several years so that early enrollees are treated and followed longer than late enrollees. In an effort to keep the contribution of individual subjects commensurate with their follow-up interval, the denominator of the incidence measure in these studies is not persons at risk for a specific time period but person-time at risk of the event. An individual followed for 10 years without becoming a case contributes 10 person-years, whereas an individual followed for 1 year contributes only one person-year to the denominator. An incidence of this type is expressed as the number of new cases per total number of person-years at risk and is sometimes called an *incidence density*.

The person-years approach is also useful for estimating the incidence of disease in large populations of known size when an accurate count of new cases and an estimate of the population at risk are available—for example, a population-based cancer registry.

A disadvantage of the incidence density approach is that it lumps together different lengths of follow-up. A small number of patients followed for a long time can contribute as much to the denominator as a large number of patients followed for a short time. If these long-term follow-up patients are systematically different from short-term follow-up patients, the resulting incidence measures may be biased.

INTERPRETING MEASURES OF CLINICAL FREQUENCY

In order to make sense of prevalence and incidence, the first step is a careful evaluation of the numerator and denominator. Two questions serve to guide this evaluation: What is a case, and what is the population?

What is a "Case"?—Defining the Numerator

Up to this point, the general term "case" has been used to indicate a disease or outcome the frequency of which is of interest. Classically, prevalence and incidence refer to the frequency of a disease among groups of people. F   ver, clinical decisions often depend on information about the frequency of disease manifestations, such as symptoms, signs, or laboratory abnormalities, or the frequency of disease effects, such as death, disability, symptomatic improvement, etc.

To interpret rates, it is necessary to know the basis upon which a case is defined, because the criteria used to define a case can strongly affect rates.

Example—One simple way to identify a case is to ask people whether they have a certain condition. How does this method compare to more rigorous methods? In the Commission on Chronic Illness study, the prevalences of various conditions, as determined by personal interviews in the home, were compared to the prevalences as determined by physician examination of the same individuals. Figure 4.2 illustrates the interview prevalences and the clinical examination prevalences for various conditions.

The data illustrate that these two methods of defining a case can generate very different estimates of prevalence and in different directions, depending on the condition (6).

For some conditions, broadly accepted, explicit diagnostic criteria are available. The American Rheumatism Association criteria for rheumatoid arthritis (Table 4.2) are an example (7). These criteria demonstrate the extraordinary specificity required to define reliably so common a disease as rheumatoid arthritis. They also illustrate a trade-off between rigorous

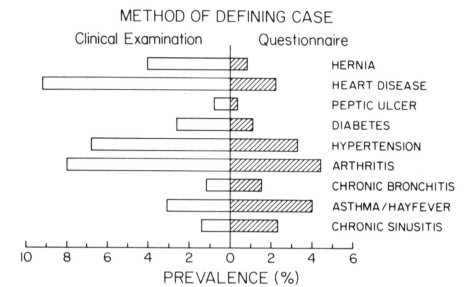

Figure 4.2. Prevalence depends on the definition of a case. The prevalence of diseases in the general population based on people's opinions (survey) and clinical evaluation. (Data from Sanders BS: Have morbidity surveys been oversold? *Am J Public Health* 52:1648–1659, 1962.

definition and clinical reality. If only "classic" cases were included in a rate, most patients who would ordinarily be considered to have the disease would not be included. On the other hand, including "probable" cases could overestimate the true rate of disease.

What is the Population?—Defining the Denominator

In order to make sense out of the number of cases, we must have a clear picture of the size and characteristics of the group of individuals in which the cases arose. A rate is useful only to the extent that the individual practitioner can decide to which kinds of patients the rate applies.

Customarily, the group indicated in the denominator of a rate is referred to as the population or, more particularly, the *population at risk*, where "at risk" means susceptible to the disease or outcome counted in the numerator. For example, it is not meaningful to describe the incidence or prevalence of cervical cancer in a population that includes women who have had hysterectomies or includes men.

Ideally, the denominator of a rate would include all people who could have the condition or a representative sample of them. But what is relevant depends on one's perspective. For example, if we wanted to know the true prevalence of rheumatoid arthritis in Americans, we would prefer to include in the denominator all people in the United States, rather than

Table 4.2
Rheumatoid Arthritis Diagnostic Criteria (American Rheumatism Association 1958 Revision)[a]

1. Morning stiffness.
2. Pain on motion or tenderness in at least one joint.[b]
3. Swelling (soft tissue thickening or fluid, not bony overgrowth alone) in at least one joint.[b]
4. Swelling of at least one other joint.[b]
5. Symmetrical joint swelling with simultaneous involvement of the same joint on both sides of the body.[b] Terminal phalangeal joint involvement will not satisfy the criterion.
6. Subcutaneous nodules over bony prominences, on extensor surfaces, or in juxta-articular regions.[b]
7. Roentgenographic changes typical of rheumatoid arthritis (which must include at least bony decalcification localized to or greatest around the involved joints and not just degenerative changes).
8. Positive agglutination (anti-gammaglobulin) test.
9. Poor mucin precipitate from synovial fluid (with shreds and cloudy solution).
10. Characteristic histologic changes in synovial membrane.
11. Characteristic histologic changes in nodules.

CATEGORIES	NUMBER OF CRITERIA REQUIRED	MINIMUM DURATION OF CONTINUOUS SYMPTOMS
Classic	7 of 11	6 weeks (Nos. 1–5)
Definite	5 of 11	6 weeks (Nos. 1–5)
Probable	3 of 11	6 weeks (1 of Nos. 1–5)

[a] Adapted from Ropes MW, Bennett CA, Cobb S, Jacox R, Jessar RA: 1958 revision of diagnostic criteria for rheumatoid arthritis. *Bull Rheum Dis* 9:175–176, 1958.
[b] Observed by physician.

patients in office practice. But if one wanted to know the prevalence of rheumatoid arthritis in office practice—perhaps in order to plan services—the relevant denominator would be patients seen in office practice, not people in the population at large. In one survey, only 25% of adults found to have arthritic and rheumatic complaints (not necessarily rheumatoid arthritis) during a community survey had received services for such complaints from any health professional or institution (8).

It is customary for epidemiologists to think of a population as consisting of all individuals residing in a geographic area. And so it should be for studies of cause-and-effect in the general population. But in studies of clinical questions, the relevant populations generally consist of patients suffering from certain diseases or exhibiting certain clinical findings, and who are found in clinical settings that are similar to those in which the information will be used. Commonly, such patients are assembled at a limited number of clinical facilities where academic physicians see patients. In these instances, the population includes all patients with the appropriate findings from the hospitals or clinics involved. They may be a small and peculiar subset of all patients with the findings in some geographic area, and even unusual for office practice in general.

What difference might the choice of a population make? What is at issue is the generalizability of observed rates. As discussed in Chapter 1, the incidence of further seizures in children who have had one febrile seizure varied from about 5% in the general population to as high as 75% in some clinics. Knowing which incidence is appropriate to one's patients is critical because it will influence the decision whether to begin chronic anticonvulsant treatment. The appropriate incidence depends upon the location and nature of the reader's practice. If the reader is an academic pediatric neurologist, referral center experience is more relevant. If the reader is a family physician or pediatrician providing community-based primary care, referral center experience may be irrelevant. Some of the authors reporting high incidences of subsequent seizures in children seen in referral centers argued that their high rate indicated that all such children should receive long-term anticonvulsant treatment. Such a conclusion may not be justified for the clinician in primary care practice, where the incidence of subsequent seizures is less than 5%.

Sampling

It is rarely possible to study all the people who have or might develop the condition of interest. Usually one takes a sample, so that the number studied is of manageable size. This raises a question: Is the sample representative of the population?

In general, there are two ways to sample. In a *random sample*, every individual in the population has an equal probability of being selected. The more general term *probability sample* is used if every person has a known (not necessarily equal) probability of being selected. On the average, the characteristics of people in probability samples are similar to those of the population from which they were selected, particularly if a large number are chosen.

Other methods of selecting samples may well be biased and so do not necessarily represent the parent population. Most groups of patients described in the medical literature, and found in most clinicians' experience, are based on biased samples. Typically, patients are included in studies because they are under care in an academic institution, available, willing to be studied, and perhaps also particularly interesting and/or severely affected. There is nothing wrong with this practice—as long as it is understood to whom the results do (or do not) apply.

RELATIONSHIP AMONG INCIDENCE, PREVALENCE, AND DURATION OF DISEASE

As described previously anything that increases the duration of the clinical findings in a patient will increase the chance that that patient will be identified in a prevalence study. The relationship among incidence and

Table 4.3

The Relationships Among Incidence, Prevalence and Duration^a of Disease: Asthma in the United States^b

AGE	ANNUAL INCIDENCE	PREVALENCE	DURATION = $\dfrac{\text{PREVALENCE}}{\text{ANNUAL INCIDENCE}}$
0–5	6/1000	29/1000	4.8 years
6–16	3/1000	32/1000	10.7 years
17–44	2/1000	26/1000	13.0 years
45–64	1/1000	33/1000	33.0 years
65+	0	36/1000	33.0 years
	3/1000	30/1000	10.0 years

^{a} Duration = $\dfrac{\text{Prevalence}}{\text{Annual Incidence}}$.

^{b} Approximated from several sources.

prevalence and duration of disease in a steady state—that is, where none of the variables is changing much over time—is approximated by the expression:

Prevalence ≈ Incidence × Average Duration of the Disease

Example—Table 4.3 shows approximate annual incidence and prevalence rates for asthma. Incidence falls with increasing age, illustrating the fact that the disease arises primarily in childhood. But prevalence stays fairly stable over the entire age span, indicating that asthma tends to be chronic and is especially chronic among older individuals. Also, because the pool of prevalent cases does not increase in size, about the same number of patients are recovering from their asthma as new patients are acquiring it.

If we use the formula (Prevalence ÷ Incidence = Average Duration), we can determine that asthma has an average duration of 10 years. When the duration of asthma is determined for each age category by dividing the prevalences by the incidences, it is apparent that the duration of asthma increases with increasing age. This reflects the clinical observation that childhood asthma often clears with time, whereas adult asthma tends to be more chronic.

BIAS IN PREVALENCE STUDIES

Prevalence studies can be used to investigate potentially causal relationships between risk factors and a disease. For this purpose, they are quick but inferior alternatives to incidence studies. Two biases are particularly troublesome: temporal sequence and old versus new cases.

Interpreting Temporal Sequences

In prevalence studies, disease and the possible factors responsible for the disease are measured simultaneously, and so it is often unclear which came before the other. The time dimension is lost, and if it is included in the interpretation it must be inferred. In contrast, studies of incidence do have

POSSIBLE CAUSES   DISEASE OR OUTCOME

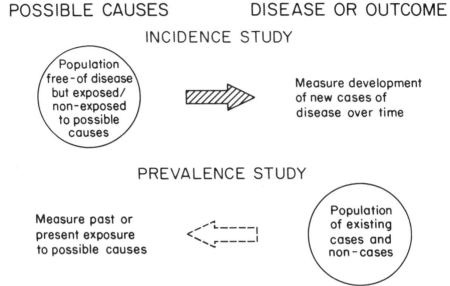

INCIDENCE STUDY

Population free-of disease but exposed/non-exposed to possible causes

Measure development of new cases of disease over time

PREVALENCE STUDY

Measure past or present exposure to possible causes

Population of existing cases and non-cases

Figure 4.3. Temporal relationship between possible causal factors and disease for incidence and prevalence studies.

a built-in sequence of events because possible causes of disease are measured initially, before disease has occurred. These relationships are illustrated in Figure 4.3.

Old Versus New Cases

The difference between cases found in the numerator of incidences and of prevalences is illustrated in Figure 4.4. In a cohort study, most new cases can be ascertained if a susceptible population is followed carefully through time. On the other hand, prevalence surveys include old as well as new cases, and they include only those cases that are available at the time of a single examination—that is, they identify only cases that happen to be both active (i.e., diagnosable) and alive at the time of the survey. Obviously, prevalences will be dominated by those patients who are able to survive their disease without losing its manifestations.

In many situations, the kinds of cases included in the numerator of an incidence are quite different from the kinds of cases included in the numerator of a prevalence. The differences may influence how the rates are interpreted.

Prevalence is affected by the average duration of disease. Rapidly fatal episodes of the disease would be included in an incidence, but most would be missed by a prevalence survey. For example, 25–40% of all deaths from coronary heart disease occur within 24 hours of the onset of symptoms in

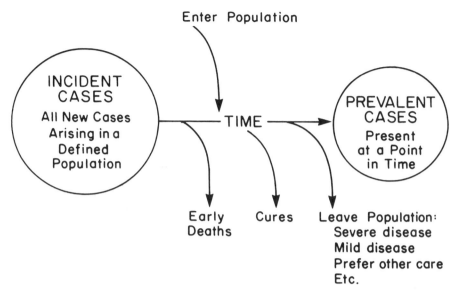

Figure 4.4. The difference in cases for incidence and prevalence studies.

individuals with no prior evidence of disease. A prevalence survey would, therefore, underestimate cases of coronary heart disease. On the other hand, diseases of long duration are well represented in prevalence surveys, even if their incidence is low. For example, although the incidence of Crohn's disease is only about 2–7/100,000/year, its prevalence is over 100/100,000, reflecting the chronic nature of the disease (9).

Prevalence surveys can also selectively include more severe cases of disease, ones that are particularly sustained and obtrusive. For example, patients with rheumatoid arthritis who are not currently active would not be included in a survey based on current symptoms and physical findings. Similarly, patients with recurrent but controllable illnesses, such as congestive heart failure or depression, may be well at a given point in time and therefore might not be discovered on a single examination. Unremitting disease, on the other hand, is less likely to be overlooked and, therefore, would contribute disproportionately to the pool of cases assembled by a prevalence survey.

USES OF INCIDENCE AND PREVALENCE

What purposes do incidence and prevalence serve? Clinicians use them in three different ways: predicting the future, describing things as they are, and making comparisons.

Predicting the Future

Incidence is a description of the rate at which a disease has arisen over time in a group of people assembled in the past. It can also be used to predict the probability that similar people will develop the condition in the future. For incidence, the sequence of events is clear because the population is known to be free of the outcome at the outset and all cases are assessed.

On the other hand, as pointed out above, prevalence describes the situation among a group of individuals at a given point in time; it offers no sound basis for predicting the future. If 30% of patients with stroke are depressed, this does not mean that 30% of stroke patients will become depressed in the future. It may be that depression predisposes to stroke or that nondepressed stroke patients are more likely to recover quickly. Because of the way in which they are measured, prevalences often reveal little about the sequence of events and only include a fraction of all possible cases. Thus, they are treacherous grounds for predicting the future.

The Probability that a Patient Has the Condition

Prevalence is particularly useful in guiding decisions about whether or not to use a diagnostic test, as pointed out in Chapter 3 because prevalence is a determinant of predictive value. Knowing that a patient with a combination of demographic and clinical characteristics has a given probability of having the disease not only influences the interpretation of a diagnostic test result but also may affect powerfully the selection among various treatment options.

The patient with pharyngitis, presented at the beginning of this chapter, illustrates how variations in prevalence can influence the approach to a clinical problem.

Example—Three approaches to the treatment of pharyngitis were compared. Their value was judged by weighing the potential benefits of preventing rheumatic fever against the costs of penicillin allergy. The three options were to obtain a throat culture and treat only those patients with throat cultures positive for β-hemolytic Group A streptococci, treat all patients without obtaining a culture, and neither culture nor treat any patient.

The analysis revealed that the optimal strategy depended upon the likelihood that a patient would have a positive culture, which can be estimated from the prevalence of streptococcal infection in the community at the time and the presence or absence of such clinical findings as fever. It was concluded that, if the probability of a positive culture for an individual patient exceeds 20%, the patient should be treated; if it is less than 5%, the patient should not be cultured or treated; and if the probability lies between 5% and 20%, the patient should be cultured first and treated based on the result (10).

This study represents a rational approach to the use of prevalences as indicators of individual probabilities of disease in guiding clinical decision making.

Making Comparisons

Although isolated incidences and prevalences serve useful functions, as described previously, they become much more powerful tools in support of clinical decisions when used to make comparisons. It is the comparison between the frequencies of disease among individuals exposed to a factor and individuals not exposed to the factor that provides the best evidence suggesting causality, not just the commonness of the disease among those exposed. For example, the risk (incidence) of lung cancer among males who smoke heavily is of the order of 0.17% per year, hardly a common event. Only when this incidence is contrasted with the incidence in nonsmokers (approximately 0.007% per year) does the devastating effect of smoking emerge. Clinicians use measures of frequency as the ingredients in comparative measures of the association between a factor and the disease or disease outcome. Ways of comparing rates will be described in more detail in Chapter 5.

SUMMARY

Most clinical questions are answered by reference to the commonness of events under varying circumstances. The commonness of clinical events is indicated by proportions or fractions, the numerators of which include the number of cases and the denominators of which include the number of people from whom the cases arose.

There are two measures of commonness—prevalence and incidence. Prevalence is the proportion of a group who have the disease at a single point in time. Incidence is the proportion of a susceptible group who develop new cases of the disease over an interval of time.

Prevalence is measured by a single survey of a group containing cases and noncases, whereas measurement of incidence requires examinations of a previously disease-free group over time. Thus, prevalence studies identify only those cases who are alive and diagnosable at the time of the survey, whereas cohort (incidence) studies ascertain all new cases. Prevalent cases, therefore, may be a biased subset of all cases because they do not include those who have already succumbed or been cured. Additionally, prevalence studies frequently do not permit a clear understanding of the temporal relationship between a causal factor and a disease.

To make sense of incidence and prevalence, the clinician must understand the basis upon which the disease is diagnosed and the characteristics of the population represented in the denominator. The latter is of particular importance in trying to decide if a given measure of incidence or prevalence pertains to patients in one's own practice.

Incidence is the most appropriate measure of commonness with which to predict the future. Prevalence serves to quantitate the likelihood that a patient with certain characteristics has the disease at a single point in time and is used for decisions about diagnosis and screening. The most powerful use of incidence and prevalence, however, is to compare different clinical alternatives.

POSTSCRIPT

Counting clinical events as described in this chapter may seem to be the most mundane of tasks. It seems so obvious that examining counts of clinical events under various circumstances is the foundation of clinical science. It may be worth reminding the reader that Pierre Louis introduced the "numerical method" of evaluating therapy less than 200 years ago. Dr. Louis had the audacity to count deaths and recoveries from febrile illness in the presence and absence of blood-letting. He was excoriated for allowing lifeless numbers to cast doubt on the healing powers of the leech, powers that had been amply confirmed by decades of astute qualitative clinical observation.

REFERENCES

1. Bryant GD, Norman GR: Expressions of probability: words and numbers. *N Engl J Med* 302:411, 1980.
2. Toogood JH: What do we mean by "usually"? *Lancet* 1:1094, 1980.
3. Friedman GD: Medical usage and abusage, "prevalence" and "incidence." *Ann Intern Med* 84:502–503, 1976.
4. O'Sullivan JB, Cathcart ES: The prevalence of rheumatoid arthritis. Follow-up evaluation of the effect of criteria on rates in Sudbury, Massachusetts. *Ann Intern Med* 76:573–577, 1972.
5. Asmundsson T, Kilburn KH: Survival after acute respiratory failure. *Ann Intern Med* 80:54–57, 1974.
6. Sanders BS: Have morbidity surveys been oversold? *Am J Publ Health* 52:1648–1659, 1962.
7. Ropes MW, Bennett GA, Cobb S, Jacox R, Jessar RA: 1958 revision of diagnostic criteria for rheumatoid arthritis. JJ Bunim (Ed). *Bull Rheum Dis* 9:175–176, 1958.
8. Spitzer WO, Harth M, Goldsmith CH, Norman GR, Dickie GL, Bass MJ, Newell JP: The arthritic complaint in primary care: prevalence, related disability, and costs. *J Rheum* 3:88–99, 1976.
9. Sedlack RE, Whisnant J, Elveback LR, Kurland LT: Incidence of Crohn's disease in Olmsted County, Minnesota, 1935–1975. *Am J Epidemiol* 112:759–763, 1980.
10. Tompkins RK, Burnes DC, Cable WE: An analysis of the cost-effectiveness of pharyngitis management and acute rheumatic fever prevention. *Ann Intern Med* 86:481–492, 1977.

SUGGESTED READINGS

Ellenberg JH, Nelson KB: Sample selection and the natural history of disease: Studies of febrile seizures. *JAMA* 243:1337–1340, 1980.
Friedman GD: Medical usage and abusage, "prevalence" and "incidence." *Ann Intern Med* 84:502–503, 1976.
Morgenstern H, Kleinbaum DG, Kupper LL: Measures of disease incidence used in epidemiologic research. *Int J Epidemiol* 9:97–104, 1980.

APPENDIX 4.1. MAIN QUESTIONS FOR DETERMINING THE VALIDITY OF STUDIES OF PREVALENCE[a]

1. What are the criteria for being a *case*?
2. What is the defined *population*?
3. Are cases and noncases from *an unbiased sample* of the population ?

[a] These questions are not meant to be all-inclusive nor to replace independent, critical thinking. They are a rough guideline, including only the most basic elements of a sound study.

chapter 5

RISK

Risk generally refers to the probability of some untoward event. In this chapter, the term "risk" is used in a more restricted sense to describe the likelihood that people who are without a disease, but are exposed to certain factors ("risk factors"), will acquire the disease.

Many people in our society have a strong interest in their risk of disease. Their concern has spawned many popular books about risk reduction and is reflected in newspaper headlines about the risk of cancer from exposure to toxic chemicals or nuclear accidents, of cardiovascular disease after use of birth control pills and of AIDS from sexual behavior or transfusion.

In this chapter, we will consider how estimates of risk are obtained by observing the relationship between exposure to possible risk factors and the subsequent incidence of disease. Then we will describe several ways of comparing risks, both as they affect individuals and populations.

RISK FACTORS

Factors that are associated with an increased risk of becoming diseased are called *risk factors*. There are several kinds of risk factors. Some, such as toxins, infectious agents, and drugs, are found in the physical environment. Others are part of the social environment. For example, disruption of family (e.g., loss of a spouse), daily routines, and culture has been shown to increase rates of disease—not only emotional but physical illness as well. Other risk factors are behavioral; among them are smoking, inactivity, and driving without seat belts. Risk factors are also inherited. For example, having the haplotype HLA B27 greatly increases the risk of acquiring the spondylarthropathies.

Exposure to a risk factor means that a person has, before becoming ill, come in contact with or has manifested the factor in question. Exposure can take place at a single point in time, as when a community is exposed to radiation during a nuclear accident. More often, however, exposure to risk factors for chronic disease takes place over a period of time. Cigarette smoking, hypertension, sexual promiscuity, and sun exposure are examples. There are many different ways of characterizing the dose of chronic exposure: ever exposed, current dose, largest dose taken, total cumulative dose, years of exposure, years since first exposure, etc. (1). Although the various measures of dose tend to be related to each other, some may show an exposure-disease relationship, whereas others do not. For example, cumulative dose of sun exposure is a risk factor for nonmelanoma skin cancer, whereas episodes of severe sunburn is a better predictor of melanoma. Choice of an appropriate measure of exposure is usually based on all that is known about the biologic effects of the exposure and the pathophysiology of the disease.

INFORMATION ABOUT RISK

Large and dramatic risks are easy for anyone to appreciate. Thus, it is not difficult to recognize the relationship between exposure and disease for such conditions as chickenpox, sunburn, or aspirin overdose because they follow exposure in a relatively rapid, certain, and obvious way. But much of the morbidity and mortality in our society is caused by chronic diseases. For these, the relationships between exposure and disease are far less obvious. It becomes virtually impossible for individual clinicians, however astute, to develop estimates of risk based on their own experiences with patients. This is true for several reasons, which are discussed below and summarized in Table 5.1.

- **Long latency**

Many chronic diseases have long latency periods between exposure to risk factors and the first manifestations of disease. Patients exposed during one time in a clinician's professional life may experience the consequences in another, years later, when the original exposure is all but forgotten. The link between exposure and disease is thereby obscured.

- **Frequent exposure to risk factors**

Many risk factors—such as cigarette smoking or driving when intoxicated—occur so frequently in our society that they scarcely seem dangerous. Only by comparing patterns of disease in other populations, or

Table 5.1
Situations in which Personal Experience is Insufficient to Establish a Relationship Between Exposure and Disease

Long latency period between exposure and disease
Frequent exposure to risk factor
Low incidence of disease
Small risk from exposure
Common disease
Multiple causes of disease

investigating special subgroups within our own (e.g., Mormons who neither smoke nor drink), can we recognize risks that are in fact rather large.

- **Low incidence of disease**
  Most diseases, even ones thought to be "common," are actually quite rare. Thus, although lung cancer is the most common kind of cancer in Americans, the yearly incidence of lung cancer even in heavy smokers is less than 2/1,000. In the average physician's practice, years may pass between new cases of lung cancer. It is difficult to draw conclusions about such infrequent events.

- **Small risk**
  If a factor confers only a small risk, a large number of "cases" are required to observe a difference in disease rates between exposed and unexposed people. This is so even if both the risk factor and the disease occur relatively frequently. It is still uncertain whether coffee and diabetes are risk factors for carcinoma of the pancreas, because estimates of risk are all small and, therefore, easily discounted as resulting from bias or chance. In contrast, it is not controversial that hepatitis B infection is a risk factor for hepatoma, because people with evidence of hepatitis B infection are hundreds of times more likely to get liver cancer than those without it.

- **Common disease**
  If the disease is one of those ordinarily occurring in our society—heart disease, cancer, or stroke—and some of the risk factors for it are already known, it becomes difficult to distinguish a new risk factor from the others. Also, there is less incentive to look for a new risk factor. For example, the syndrome of sudden, unexpected death in adults is a common way to die. Many cases seem related to coronary heart disease. However, it is entirely conceivable that there are other important causes, as yet unrecognized because an adequate explanation for most cases is available.

  On the other hand, rare diseases invite efforts to find a cause. Phocomelia is such an unusual congenital malformation that the appearance of just a few cases raised suspicion that some new agent (as it turned out, the drug, thalidomide) might be responsible. Similarly, physicians were quick to notice when several cases of carcinoma of the vagina, a very rare condition, began appearing. A careful search for an explanation was undertaken, and maternal exposure to diethylstilbestrol was found.

- **Multiple causes and effects**
  There is usually not a close, one-to-one, relationship between a risk factor and one particular disease. Some people with hypertension develop congestive heart failure and many do not. Many people who do not have hypertension develop congestive heart failure as well. The relationship between hypertension and congestive heart failure is obscured by the fact that there are several other causes of the disease, and hypertension causes several diseases. Thus, although people with hypertension are about three times more likely to develop congestive heart failure and hypertension is

the leading cause of that condition, physicians were not particularly attuned to this relationship until recently, when adequate data became available.

For these reasons, individual clinicians are rarely in a position to confirm associations between exposure and disease, though they may suspect them. For accurate information, they must turn to the medical literature, particularly studies that are carefully constructed and involve a large number of patients.

USES OF RISK

Information about risk serves several purposes.

Prediction

Risk factors are used, first and foremost, to predict the occurrence of disease. The quality of predictions depends on the similarity of the people on whom the estimate is based to the people for whom the prediction is made.

Although risk factors may signify an individual's increased risk of disease, relative to an unexposed person, their presence does not mean that an individual is very likely to get the disease. Most people, even those with many strong risk factors, are unlikely to get a disease—at least over several years' time. Thus, a heavy cigarette smoker, who has a twenty-fold increase in the risk of lung cancer compared to nonsmokers, nevertheless has only a one in a hundred chance of getting lung cancer in the next 10 years.

In individual patients, risk factors usually are not as strong predictors of disease as are clinical findings of early disease. As Rose put it:

Often the best predictor of future major diseases is the presence of existing minor disease. A low ventilatory function today is the best predictor of its future rate of decline. A high blood pressure today is the best predictor of its future rate of rise. Early coronary heart disease is better than all of the conventional risk factors as a predictor of future fatal disease (2).

Cause

It is often assumed that any excess incidence of disease in exposed versus nonexposed persons is because of exposure to a risk factor. However, risk factors need not be causes. A risk factor may mark a disease outcome indirectly, by virtue of an association with some other determinant(s) of disease—that is, it may be confounded with a causal factor. For example, lack of maternal education is a risk factor for low birth weight infants. Yet, other factors related to education, such as poor nutrition, less prenatal care, cigarette smoking, etc., are more directly the causes of low birth weight.

A risk factor that is not a cause of disease is called a *marker*, because it "marks" the increased probability of disease. Not being a cause does not diminish the value of a risk factor as a way of predicting the probability of disease. But it does imply that removing such a risk factor might not remove the excess risk associated with it.

Diagnosis

The presence of a risk factor increases the probability that a disease is present. Knowledge of risk, therefore, can be used in the diagnostic process, inasmuch as increasing the prevalence of disease among patients tested is one way of improving the performance (positive predictive value) of a diagnostic test.

However, the presence of a risk factor usually increases the probability of disease very little for any one individual at one point in time, compared to other aspects of the clinical situation. For example, age and sex are relatively strong risk factors for coronary artery disease, yet the prevalence of disease in the most at-risk age and sex group, old men, is only 12.3% compared to 0.4% for the least at-risk group, young women. When specifics of the clinical situation, such as type of chest pain and results of an electrocardiographic stress test, are considered as well, the prevalence of coronary disease can be raised to 99.8% for old men and 93.1% for young women (3).

More often, it is helpful to use the absence of a risk factor to help rule out disease, particularly when one factor is strong and predominant. Thus, it would be reasonable to consider mesothelioma in the differential diagnosis of a pleural mass if the patient were an asbestos worker; but mesothelioma would be considerably less likely if the patient had never worked with asbestos. Knowledge of risk factors is also used to improve the efficiency of screening programs by selecting subgroups of patients at increased risk.

Prevention

If a risk factor is also a cause of disease, its removal can be used to prevent disease whether or not the mechanism by which the disease takes place is known. Some of the classic events in the history of epidemiology are illustrations. For example, before bacteria were identified Snow found an increased rate of cholera among people drinking water supplied by a particular company and controlled an epidemic by cutting off that supply. The concept of cause and its relationship to prevention will be discussed in Chapter 11.

PROBABILITY AND THE INDIVIDUAL

The best available information for predicting disease in an individual is past experience with a large number of similar people. For example, an observed incidence of 2/1000/year for the occurrence of lung cancer in heavy smokers becomes an estimate of the probability, 0.002, that an individual heavy smoker will get lung cancer in a year. In practical terms, incidence is used to estimate the probability that an individual will experience the event of interest. If our knowledge of human disease were more complete, we would not need to resort to probability. But we do not have that luxury.

However, there is a basic incompatibility between the incidence of a disease in groups of people and chances that an individual will contract that disease. Quite naturally, both patients and clinicians would like to answer questions about the future occurrence of disease as precisely as possible. They are uncomfortable about assigning a probability, such as the chances that a person will get lung cancer or stroke in the next 5 years. Moreover, any one person will, at the end of 5 years, either have the disease or not. So in a sense, the average is always wrong for the individual, because it is expressed in different terms.

Nevertheless, probabilities can guide clinical decision making. Even if a prediction does not come true in an individual patient, it will usually be borne out in many such cases. After all, weather forecasts are not always accurate either, but they do help us decide whether to carry an umbrella.

STUDIES OF RISK

There are several scientific strategies for determining risk. In general, there is a trade-off between scientific rigor and feasibility.

Observational Studies

The most satisfactory way of determining whether exposure to a potential risk factor results in an increased risk of disease would be to conduct an experiment. People currently without disease would be divided into groups of equal susceptibility to the disease in question. One group would be exposed to the purported risk factor and the other would not, but the groups would otherwise be treated the same. Later, any difference in observed rates of disease in the groups could be attributed to the risk factor.

Unfortunately, the effects of most risk factors cannot be studied in this way. Consider some of the questions of risk that concern us today. Are inactive people at increased risk for cardiovascular disease, everything else being equal? Does heterosexual exposure lead to AIDS? Do seat belts decrease the risk of dying from an auto accident? For such questions as these, it is usually not possible to conduct an experiment. People become exposed or not to risk factors for reasons that have nothing to do with the scientific value of the information their exposure may provide. As a result, it is usually necessary to study risk in less obtrusive ways.

Clinical studies in which the researcher gathers data by simply observing events as they happen, without playing an active part in what takes place, are called *observational studies*. On the other hand, in *experimental studies*, the researcher determines who is exposed. Although experimental studies are more scientifically rigorous, observational studies are the only feasible way of studying most questions of risk.

Observational studies are subject to a great many more potential biases than are experiments. When people become exposed or not exposed to a certain risk factor in the natural course of events, they are also likely to differ in a great many other ways. If these ways are also related to disease they could account for any association observed between risk factors and disease.

This leads to the main challenge of observational studies: to deal with extraneous differences between exposure groups in order to mimic as closely as possible an experiment. The differences are considered "extraneous" from the point of view of someone trying to determine cause-effect relationships. The following example illustrates one approach to handling such differences.

Example—Although the presence of sickle-cell trait (HbAS) is generally regarded as a benign condition, several studies have suggested that it is associated with defects in physical growth and cognitive development. A study was undertaken, therefore, to see if children born with HbAS experienced problems in growth and development more frequently than children with normal hemoglobin (HbAA), everything else being equal. It was recognized that a great many other factors are related both to growth and development and also to having HbAS. Among these are race, sex, birth date, birth weight, gestational age, 5-minute Apgar score, and socioeconomic status. If these were not taken into account, it would not be possible to distinguish the effects of HbAS, in and of itself, from the effects of the other factors. The authors chose to deal with these other factors by matching. For each child with HbAS, they selected a child with HbAA who was similar with respect to the seven other factors. Fifty newborns with HbAS and 50 with HbAA were followed from birth to 3–5 years old. No differences in growth and development were found (4).

Other ways of dealing with differences between groups will be described in the next chapter (Chapter 6).

Cohorts

The term *cohort* is used to describe a group of people who have something in common when they are first assembled, and who are then observed for a period of time to see what happens to them. Table 5.2 lists some of the ways in which cohorts are used in clinical research.

Whatever members of a cohort have in common, observations of them should fulfill two criteria if they are to provide sound information.

First, cohorts should be observed over a meaningful period of time in the natural history of the disease in question. This is so there will be sufficient time for the risk to be expressed. If we wish to learn whether neck irradiation during childhood results in thyroid neoplasms, a 5-year follow-up would not be a fair test of the risk associated with irradiation, because the usual time period between exposure and the onset of this disease is considerably longer.

Second, all members of the cohort should be observed over the full

Table 5.2
Cohorts and their Purposes

CHARACTERISTIC IN COMMON	TO ASSESS EFFECT OF	EXAMPLE
Age	Age	Life expectancy for people age 70 (regardless of when born)
Date of birth	Calendar time	Tuberculosis rates for people born in 1910
Exposure	Risk factor	Lung cancer in people who smoke
Disease	Prognosis	Survival rate for patients with breast cancer
Preventive intervention	Prevention	Reduction in incidence of pneumonia after pneumococcal vaccination
Therapeutic intervention	Treatment	Improvement in survival for patients with Hodgkin's disease given combination chemotherapy

period of follow-up. To the extent that people drop out of the cohort and their reasons for dropping out are related in some way to the outcome, the information provided by an incomplete cohort can be a distortion of the true state of affairs.

Cohort Studies

In a *cohort study*, a group of people (a cohort) is assembled, none of whom has experienced the outcome of interest. On entry to the study, people in the cohort are classified according to those characteristics that might be related to outcome. These people are then observed over time to see which of them experience the outcome. It is then possible to see how initial characteristics relate to subsequent outcome events. A cohort study is diagrammed in Figure 5.1. Other names for such studies are *longitudinal* (emphasizing that patients are followed over time), *prospective* (implying the forward direction in which the patients are pursued), and *incidence* (calling attention to the basic measure of new disease events over time).

The following is a description of a classical cohort study, which has made an extremely important contribution to our understanding of cardiovascular disease.

Example—The Framingham Study was begun in 1949 to identify factors associated with an increased risk of coronary heart disease (CHD). A representative sample of 5209 men and women, aged 30–59, was selected from approximately 10,000 persons of that age living in Framingham, a small town near Boston. Of these, 5127 were free of CHD when first examined and, therefore, were at risk of

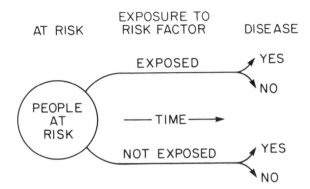

AT RISK
EXPOSURE TO
RISK FACTOR
DISEASE

EXPOSED → YES
↘ NO

PEOPLE
AT
RISK
— TIME →

NOT EXPOSED → YES
↘ NO

Figure 5.1.   Design of a cohort study of risk.

developing CHD subsequently. These people have been re-examined biennially for evidence of coronary disease. The study has run for 30 years and has demonstrated that risk of developing CHD is associated with blood pressure, serum cholesterol, cigarette smoking, glucose intolerance, and left ventricular hypertrophy. There is a large difference in risk between those with none and those with all of these risk factors (5).

Historical Cohort Studies

Cohort studies can be conducted in two ways (Fig. 5.2). The cohort can be assembled in the present and followed into the future (a *concurrent cohort study*); or it can be identified from past records and followed forward from that time up to the present (a *historical cohort study*).

Most of the advantages and disadvantages of cohort studies, as a strategy, apply whether they are concurrent or historical. However, the potential for difficulties with the quality of data is different for the two. In concurrent studies, data can be collected specifically for the purposes of the study and with full anticipation of what is needed. It is thereby possible to avoid biases that might undermine the accuracy of the data. On the other hand, data for historical cohorts are often gathered for other purposes—usually as part of medical records for patient care. These data may not be of sufficient quality for rigorous research.

Disadvantages of Cohort Studies

Cohort studies of risk are the best available substitute for a true experiment, when experimentation is not possible. However, they present a considerable number of practical difficulties of their own. Some of the advantages and disadvantages of cohort studies, for the purpose of describing risk factors, are summarized in Table 5.3.

The principal disadvantage is that, if the outcome is infrequent, and most are, a large number of people must be entered in a study and remain under observation for a long time before results are available. For example,

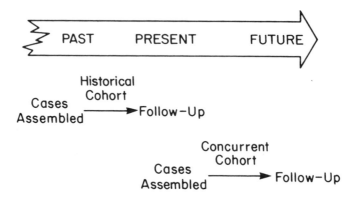

Figure 5.2. Historical and concurrent cohort studies.

Table 5.3
Advantages and Disadvantages of Cohort Studies

ADVANTAGES	DISADVANTAGES
The only way of establishing incidence (i.e., absolute risk) directly	Inefficient, because many more subjects must be enrolled than experience the event of interest; therefore, cannot be used for rare diseases
Follow the same logic as the clinical question: if persons exposed, then do they get the disease?	Expensive because of resources necessary to study many people over time
Exposure can be elicited without the bias that might occur if outcome were already known	Results not available for a long time
Can assess the relationship between exposure and many diseases	Can only assess the relationship between disease and of exposure to relatively few factors (i.e., those recorded at the outset of the study)

the Framingham Study of coronary heart disease was the largest of its kind and studied one of the most frequent of the chronic diseases in America. Nevertheless, over 5000 people had to be followed for several years before the first, preliminary conclusions could be published. Only 5% of the people had experienced a coronary event during the first 8 years!

A related problem with cohort studies results from the fact that the people being studied are usually "free living" and not under the control of researchers. A great deal of effort and money must be expended to keep track of them. Cohort studies, therefore, are expensive, sometimes costing millions of dollars.

Because of the time and money required for cohort studies, this approach cannot be used for all clinical questions about risk. For practical reasons, the cohort approach has been reserved for only the most important questions. This has led to efforts to find more efficient, yet dependable ways of assessing risk. One of these ways, case control studies, will be discussed in Chapter 10.

COMPARING RISKS

The basic expression of risk is incidence, defined in Chapter 4 as the number of new cases of disease arising in a defined population during a given period of time. But usually we want to compare the incidence of disease in two or more cohorts, which have different exposures to some possible risk factor. To compare risks, several measures of the association between exposure and disease, called *measures of effect*, are commonly used. They represent different concepts of risk and are used for different purposes. Four measures of effect are discussed below, summarized in Table 5.4, and illustrated by an example in Table 5.5.

Attributable Risk

First, one might ask, "What is the additional risk (incidence) of disease following exposure, over and above that experienced by people who are not exposed?" The answer is expressed as *attributable risk*, the incidence of disease in exposed persons minus the incidence in nonexposed persons. Attributable risk is the additional incidence of disease related to exposure, taking into account the background incidence of disease, presumably from other causes. Note that this way of comparing rates implies that the risk factor is a cause and not just a marker. Because of the way it is calculated, attributable risk is also called *risk difference*.

Table 5.4
Measures of Effect

EXPRESSION	QUESTION	DEFINITION[a]
Attributable risk (risk difference)	What is the incidence of disease attributable to exposure?	$AR = I_E - I_{\bar{E}}$
Relative risk (risk ratio)	How many times more likely are exposed persons to become diseased, relative to nonexposed?	$RR = \dfrac{I_E}{I_{\bar{E}}}$
Population attributable risk	What is the incidence of disease in a population, associated with the occurrence of a risk factor?	$AR_p = AR \times P$
Population attributable fraction	What fraction of disease in a population is attributable to exposure to a risk factor?	$AF_P = \dfrac{AR_p}{I_T}$

[a] Where:
  I_E = incidence in exposed persons
  $I_{\bar{E}}$ = incidence in nonexposed persons
  P = prevalence of exposure to a risk factor
  I_T = total incidence of disease in a population

Table 5.5
Calculating Measures of Effect: Cigarette Smoking and Death from Lung Cancer[a]

Simple Risks	
Death rate from lung cancer in cigarette smokers	0.96/1000/year
Death rate from lung cancer in nonsmokers	0.07/1000/year
Prevalence of cigarette smoking	56%
Total death rate from lung cancer	0.56/1000/year

Compared Risks
Attributable risk = 0.96/1000/year − 0.07/1000/year
= 0.89/1000/year

$$\text{Relative risk} = \frac{0.96/1000/\text{year}}{0.07/1000/\text{year}}$$
= 13.7

Population attributable risk = 0.89/1000/year × 0.56
= 0.50/1000/year

$$\text{Population attributable fraction} = \frac{0.50/1000/\text{year}}{0.56/1000/\text{year}}$$
= 0.89

[a] Estimated data from Doll R, Hill AB: *Br Med J* 1:1399–1410, 1964.

Relative Risk

On the other hand, one might ask, "How many times more likely are exposed persons to get the disease relative to nonexposed persons?" To answer this question, we speak of *relative risk* or *risk ratio*, the ratio of incidence in exposed persons to incidence in nonexposed persons. Relative risk tells us nothing about the magnitude of absolute risk (incidence). Even for large relative risks, the absolute risk might be quite small if the disease is uncommon. It does tell us the strength of the association between exposure and disease and so is a useful measure of effect for studies of disease etiology.

Interpreting Estimates of Individual Risk

The clinical meaning attached to relative and attributable risk is often quite different, because the two expressions of risk stand for entirely different concepts. The appropriate expression of risk depends upon the question being asked.

Example—The Royal College of General Practitioners has been conducting a study of the health effects of oral contraceptives. During 1968 and 1969, over 23,000 women taking oral contraceptives and an equal number of women who had never taken the pill were entered into the study by 1400 physicians. These physicians subsequently reported oral contraceptive use, morbidity, and mortality twice a year. The use of oral contraceptives was updated regularly. After 10 years of follow-

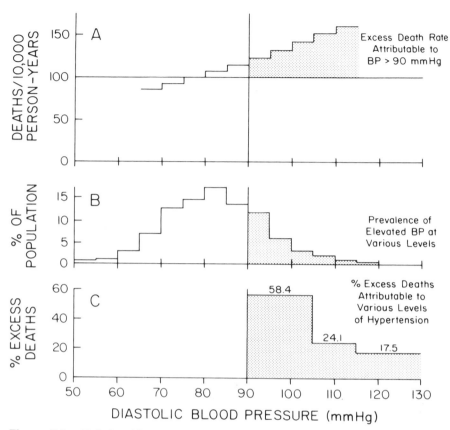

Figure 5.3.   Relationships among attributable risk, prevalence of risk factor, and population risk for hypertension. (Adapted from The Hypertension Detection and Follow-up Cooperative Group. *Ann NY Acad Sci,* 304:254–266, 1978.)

up, it was reported that oral contraceptive users had a risk of dying from circulatory diseases that was 4.2 times greater than for nonusers. But the risk of dying was increased by only 22.7/100,000 women-years. An individual woman, weighing the risks of oral contraceptives, must deal with the two concepts of risk very differently. On the one hand, a four-fold greater risk of dying might loom large. On the other, two chances in 10,000 is a very remote possibility (6).

In general, because attributable risk represents the actual, additional probability of disease in those exposed, it is a more meaningful expression of risk in most clinical situations.

Population Risk

Another way of looking at risk is to ask, "How much does a risk factor contribute to the overall rates of disease in groups of people, rather than individuals?" This information is useful for deciding which risk factors are particularly important and which are trivial to the overall health of a community, and so it can inform those in policy positions how to choose priorities for the deployment of health care resources.

To estimate population risk, it is necessary to take into account the frequency with which members of a community are exposed to a risk factor. A relatively weak risk factor (in terms of relative risk) that is quite prevalent could account for more of the overall incidence of disease in a community than a stronger risk factor that is rarely present.

Population attributable risk is a measure of the excess incidence of disease in a community that is associated with the occurrence of a risk factor. It is the product of the attributable risk and the prevalence of the risk factor in a population.

One can also describe the fraction of disease occurrence in a population that is associated with a particular risk factor, the *population attributable fraction*. It is obtained by dividing the population attributable risk by the total incidence of disease in the population.

Figure 5.3 illustrates how the prevalence of a risk factor determines the relationship between individual and population risk. *A* shows the attributable risk of death according to diastolic blood pressure. Risk increases with increasing blood pressure. However, few people have extremely high blood pressure (*B*). When hypertension is taken to be a diastolic blood pressure ≥ 90 mm Hg, most hypertensive people are just over 90 and very few are in the highest category, 115 mm Hg. As a result (*C*), the greatest percentage of excess deaths in the population (58.4%), is attributable to relatively low-grade hypertension, 90–105 mm Hg. Paradoxically, then, physicians could save more lives by effective treatment of mild hypertension than severe hypertension.

Measures of population risk are less frequently encountered in the clinical literature than are measures of individual risk, e.g., attributable and relative risk. But a particular practice is as much a population for its health care providers as is a community for health policy makers. Also, the concept of how the prevalence of exposure affects risk in groups can be important in the care of individual patients. For instance, when patients cannot give a history or when exposure is difficult for them to recognize, we depend on the usual prevalence of exposure to estimate the likelihood of various diseases. When considering treatable causes of cirrhosis in a North American patient, for example, it would be more profitable to consider alcohol than schistosomes, inasmuch as few North Americans are exposed to *Schistosoma mansoni*. Of course, one might take a very different stance in the Nile Delta, where people rarely drink alcohol and schistosomes are prevalent.

SUMMARY

Risk factors are characteristics that are associated with an increased risk of becoming diseased. Whether or not a particular risk factor is a cause of disease, its presence allows one to predict the probability that disease will occur.

Most suspected risk factors cannot be manipulated for the purposes of an experiment, so it is usually necessary to study risk by simply observing people's experience with risk factors and disease. One way of doing so is to select a cohort of people who are and are not exposed to a risk factor and observe their subsequent incidence of disease.

When disease rates are compared, the results can be expressed in several ways. Attributable risk is the excess incidence of disease related to exposure. Relative risk is the number of times more likely exposed people are to become diseased, relative to nonexposed. The impact of a risk factor on groups of people takes into account not only the risk related to exposure but the prevalence of exposure as well.

Although it is scientifically preferable to study risk by means of cohort studies, this approach is not always feasible because of the time, effort, and expense they entail.

REFERENCES

1. Weiss NS, Liff JM: Accounting for the multicausal nature of disease in the design and analysis of epidemiologic studies. *Am J Epidemiol* 117:14–18, 1983.
2. Rose G: Sick individuals and sick populations. *Int J Epidemiol* 14:32–38, 1985.
3. Diamond GA, Forrester JS: Analysis of probability as an aid in the clinical diagnosis of coronary-artery disease. *N Engl J Med* 300:1350–1358, 1979.
4. Kramer MS, Rooks Y, Pearson HA: Growth and development in children with sickle-cell trait. *N Engl J Med* 299:686–689, 1978.
5. Dawber TR: *The Framingham Study. The Epidemiology of Atherosclerotic Disease.* Cambridge, Harvard University Press, 1980.
6. Royal College of General Practitioners' Oral Contraception Study: Further analysis of mortality in oral contraceptive users. *Lancet* 1:541–546, 1981.

SUGGESTED READINGS

Dawber TR: *The Framingham Study. The Epidemiology of Atherosclerotic Disease.* Cambridge, Harvard University Press, 1980.
Morganstern H, Kleinbaum DG, Kupper LL: Measures of disease incidence used in epidemiologic research. *Int J Epidemiol* 9:97–104, 1980.
Relative or attributable risk? Editorial. *Lancet* 2:1211–1212, 1981.
Rose G: Sick individuals and sick populations. *Int J Epidemiol* 14:32–38, 1985.

chapter **6**

PROGNOSIS

When people become sick, they have a great many questions about how their illness will affect them. Is it dangerous? Could I die of it? Will there be pain? How long will I be able to continue my present activities? Will it ever go away altogether? Most patients want to know what to expect; regardless of whether anything can be done about their illness.

Prognosis is a prediction of the future course of disease following its onset. In this chapter, we review the ways in which the course of disease can be described. We will then consider the biases that can affect these descriptions and how these biases can be controlled. Our intention is to give readers a better understanding of a difficult but indispensable task: predicting patients' futures as closely as possible. The object is to avoid expressing prognosis with vagueness when it is unnecessary, and with certainty when it is misleading.

DIFFERENCES BETWEEN RISK AND PROGNOSIS

Although risk and prognosis have many similarities and both are assessed by means of cohort studies, a distinction should be made between conditions that increase the risk of getting a disease and those that predict the course once the disease is present. The former, as discussed in Chapter 5, are called risk factors: conditions that can be identified in well persons and, when present, are associated with an increased risk of acquiring disease. The latter are called *prognostic factors:* conditions that, when present in persons already known to have disease, are associated with an outcome of the disease.

Risk and prognosis fall along the same continuum in the course of disease. Why consider them separately? We touched on this question in the preceding chapter and will elaborate here.

Difference in Rates

First, risk factors generally predict low probability events. Yearly rates for the onset of various diseases are in the order of 1/100 to 1/10,000. As a result, relationships between exposure and risk usually elude even astute clinicians unless they rely on carefully executed studies, often involving a large number of subjects over an extended period of time. Prognosis, on the other hand, describes relatively frequent events. Clinicians can form some sort of estimate of prognosis on their own, from their personal experience. Of course, these estimates can be more or less precise, depending on the methods used.

Differences in Outcomes

Risk and prognosis describe different phenomena. For risk, the event being counted is the onset of disease. For prognosis, a variety of consequences of disease are counted, including death, complications, disability, suffering, etc. These events will be considered later in this chapter.

Differences in Risk and Prognostic Factors

Factors associated with an increased risk are not necessarily the same as those marking a worse prognosis and are often considerably different for a given disease. For example, low blood pressure decreases one's chances of having an acute myocardial infarction, but is a bad prognostic sign when present during an acute event (Fig. 6.1). Similarly, intake of exogenous estrogens during menopause increases women's risk of endometrial cancer, but the associated cancers are found at an earlier stage and seem to have a better-than-average prognosis.

Some factors do have a similar effect on both risk and prognosis. Men are more likely than women to acquire coronary disease in middle age and are also more likely to die if they get it. Also, both the risk of experiencing an acute myocardial infarction and the risk of dying of it increase with age.

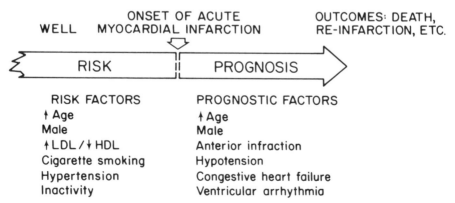

Figure 6.1. Differences between risk and prognostic factors for acute myocardial infarction.

NATURAL HISTORY/CLINICAL COURSE

Natural History

The *natural history* of disease is the evolution of disease without medical intervention; that is, how patients will fare if nothing is done for their disease.

Is it practical even to ask about natural history in countries where medical care is widely sought after and available? That depends on the disease. A great many diseases generally do not come under medical care during a large part of their course, if at all. They remain unrecognized, perhaps because they are asymptomatic or are considered among the ordinary discomforts of daily living. Mild depression, anemia, and cancers that are occult and slow growing (e.g., some cancers of the thyroid and prostate) are examples of such diseases.

Clinical Course

There are other diseases for which patients regularly come under medical care at some time in the course of their illness. These diseases tend to assume a high profile because they cause symptoms such as pain, failure to thrive, disfigurement, or unusual behavior, that compel patients or their families to seek care. Examples include type I diabetes mellitus, carcinoma of the lung, and rabies. Once disease is recognized, it is also likely to be treated. The term *clinical course* has been used to describe the evolution of disease that has come under medical care and is then treated in a variety of ways that might affect the subsequent course of events.

Sampling Bias

Descriptions of the course of disease report on samples and so are susceptible to a sampling bias.

Published accounts of disease that are based on experience in special centers can paint a misleading picture of the disease in less selected patients. The recognized cases may be particularly severely affected or may have come to attention because the patients had other symptoms that were not related to the disease in question. Therefore, it is important to ask just how natural the history observed is. The true natural history of unselected cases of a disease, and the course of those that are recognized, can be quite different.

Example—Hereditary spherocytosis (HS) is a defect of red cell membranes that is inherited as an autosomal dominant trait. In its classical form, HS is characterized by hemolytic anemia and splenomegaly; the presence of spherical red cells can be seen on blood smears. Usually production of red cells keeps pace with hemolysis, but anemia can be severe if production is reduced for some reason, such as acute infection or old age. A definitive diagnosis can be made by testing red cells for osmotic fragility.

Although some people with HS are severely affected, a great many others are asymptomatic. Having no reasons to consult physicians or to have special tests done, they generally escape detection and so contribute little to our picture of the usual course of HS. This should be borne in mind when counseling patients who are well and are discovered to have HS only because they were screened, after a relative was found to have the disease.

Even for diseases that regularly come under care, prognoses reported in the medical literature may be systematically different from the usual course of disease, as pointed out in Chapter 1. Most academic physicians' experience and most published reports come from medical centers, and patients seen in medical centers are usually not a representative sample of patients who are in the community and cared for by local physicians. In fact, the reasons for referral are often related to prognosis. Many patients are sent because they are doing badly. Perhaps the usual treatments have been given and have not worked. Sometimes the patient has an unusual or perplexing complication of disease or other features that suggest trouble is brewing. Under these circumstances, both patients and physicians may want to seek more expert opinion.

The following is an example of how sampling bias can affect our understanding of prognosis.

Example—Multiple sclerosis (MS) seems to be a crippling and lethal disease when seen from the perspective of neurology clinics and hospitals. However, when the clinical course of MS is described for all patients developing the disease in a defined geographic region, a different picture emerges. In one such study (Fig. 6.2) one-half of the patients were alive 50 years after onset, about the same number as would have been expected for people of the same age and sex who did not have MS. Most patients were alive and ambulatory 10 years after diagnosis (1).

As a general rule, reports of prognosis based on experience in academic

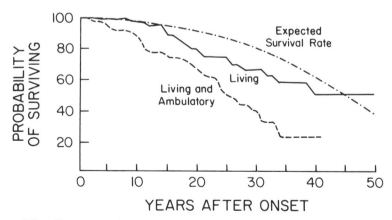

Figure 6.2. Prognosis of disease in a community: survival and mobility after the onset of multiple sclerosis. (Redrawn from Percy AK, Nobrega FT, Okazaki H, Glattre E, Kurland LT: *Arch Intern Med* 25:105–111, 1971.)

medical centers cannot be taken as an accurate guide to prognosis in less selected medical settings. Usually, reported cases will have a worse-than-average prognosis.

DESCRIBING OUTCOMES OF DISEASE

Descriptions of prognosis should include the full range of manifestations that would be considered important to patients. By this is meant not only death and disease, but also consequences of disease, such as pain, anguish, and inability to care for one's self or pursue usual activities.

In their efforts to be "scientific," physicians sometimes value certain kinds of outcomes over others, at the expense of clinical relevance. Clinical effects that cannot be directly perceived by patients—for example, reduction in tumor size, normalization of blood chemistries, or change in serology—are not ends in themselves. These biologic phenomena can be substituted for clinical outcomes only if the two are known to be related to each other. Thus, hypercalcemia is an important clinical outcome of hyperparathyroidism only if it causes such symptoms as drowsiness or thirst or if there is reason to believe that it will eventually lead to complication, such as bone or kidney disease. If an outcome cannot be related to something patients will recognize, the information should not be used to guide patient care, although it may be of considerable value in understanding the origins and mechanisms of disease.

Table 6.1 provides a view of how outcomes are described to physicians in the general medical literature. It is apparent that authors of research articles are particularly fond of "hard," biologic data, of the sort provided by diagnostic tests. On the other hand, outcomes of even greater importance to patients, such as the ability to carry on daily activities, receive short shrift, even in reports of prognosis or the effects of treatment, where such outcomes are clinically important. At best, the medical literature does not provide much information about some important outcomes of disease. At worst, it may change the reader's perceptions about what is important in clinical medicine.

Table 6.1
Outcomes of Disease Reported in the Medical Literature[a]

OUTCOME	PERCENTAGE OF ARTICLES
Diagnostic Tests	90
Physical Signs	68
Symptoms	63
Death	18
Social or Occupational Function	3
Mental Status	1

[a] For N Engl J Med, JAMA, and Lancet, 1976. From Fletcher RH, Fletcher SW: N Engl J Med 301:180–183, 1979.

Zero Time

Cohorts are observed starting from a point in time, called *zero time*. This point should be specified clearly and be the same, well-defined location along the course of disease—for example, the onset of symptoms, time of diagnosis, beginning of treatment—for each patient. For studies of prognosis, the term *inception cohort* is used to describe a group of people who are assembled near the onset ("inception") of disease.

If observation is begun at different points in the course of disease for the various patients in the cohort, description of their subsequent course will lack precision. The relative timing of such events as recovery, recurrence, or death would be difficult to interpret or misleading.

For example, suppose we wanted to describe the clinical course of patients with lung cancer. We would assemble a cohort of people with the disease and follow them forward over time to such outcomes as complications and death. But what do we mean by "with disease"? If zero time was detection by screening for some patients, onset of symptoms for others, and hospitalization or the beginning of treatment for still others, then observed prognosis would depend on the particular mix of zero times in the study. Worse, if we did not explicitly describe when in the course of disease patients entered the cohort, we would not know how to interpret or use the reported prognosis at all.

PROGNOSIS AS A RATE

It is convenient to summarize the course of disease as a single number. Rates commonly used for this purpose are shown in Table 6.2. These rates have in common the same basic components of incidence: events arising in a cohort of patients over time (Chapter 4).

All the components of the rate must be specified: zero time, people at risk, definition of events, and time of follow-up. If the interval of follow-up is not specified, it must be long enough for all the events to occur.

Table 6.2
Rates Commonly Used to Describe Prognosis

RATE	DEFINITION
Five-year survival	Percent of patients surviving 5 years from some point in the course of their disease
Case-fatality	Percent of patients with a disease who die of it[a]
Response	Percent of patients showing some evidence of improvement following an intervention[a]
Remission	Percent of patients entering a phase in which disease is no longer detectable[a]
Recurrence	Percent of patients who have return of disease after a disease-free interval[a]

[a] Time under observation is either stated or assumed to be sufficiently long so that all events that will occur have been observed.

Otherwise, the observed "rate" (proportion of people experiencing the event) will understate the true one.

A Tradeoff: Simplicity versus Loss of Information

Expressing prognosis as a rate has the virtue of simplicity. Rates can be committed to memory and communicated succinctly. Their drawback is that very little information is conveyed, so that vast differences in prognosis can be hidden within similar summary rates.

Figure 6.3 shows 5-year survival for patients with four conditions. For each condition, about 10% of the patients are alive at 5 years. But the summary rate, 10% survival, fails to express differences of considerable importance. In *A*, patients with lung cancer presenting as a solitary pul-

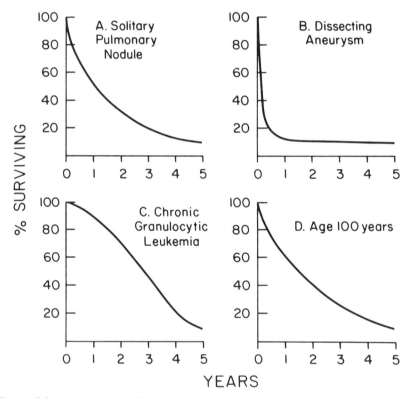

Figure 6.3. A limitation of 5-year survival rates: four conditions with the same 5-year survival rate of 10%. (Data from Steele JD: *The Solitary Pulmonary Nodule.* Springfield, IL. Charles C Thomas, 1964; Anagnostopoulos CE, Manakavalan JS, Prabhaker MD, Kittle CF: *Am J Cardiology* 30:263–273, 1972; Kardinal CG, Bateman JR, Weiner J: *Arch Intern Med* 136:305–313, 1976; and *1979 Life Insurance Fact Book.* Washington, DC, American College of Life Insurance, 1979.)

monary nodule die more rapidly at first than they do later, suggesting that the tumors are responsible for early death, after which the risk associated with the tumor falls off. *B* shows that patients with dissecting aneurysm experience a huge mortality early on; but if they survive the first few months, their risk of dying is not affected by having had the dissection. Chronic myelocytic leukemia (*C*) is a condition that has relatively little effect on survival during the first few years after diagnosis. Later, there is an acceleration in mortality rate until nearly all patients are dead 5 years after diagnosis. *D* is presented as a benchmark. Only at age 100 do people in the general population have a 5-year survival rate comparable to that of patients with the three diseases.

Survival Analysis

When interpreting prognosis, we would like to know the likelihood, on the average, that patients with a given condition will experience an outcome at any point in time. When prognosis is expressed as a summary rate it does not contain this information. However, there are methods for presenting information about average time-to-event for any time in the course of disease.

"Survival" of a Cohort

The most straightforward way to learn about survival is to assemble a cohort of patients with the condition at some point in the course of their illness (e.g., onset of symptoms, diagnosis, or beginning of treatment) and keep them under observation until all could have experienced the outcome of interest. For a small cohort, one might then represent the experience with these patients' course of disease as shown in Figure 6.4A. The plot of survival against time displays steps, corresponding to the death of each of the ten patients in the cohort. If the number of patients were increased (Fig. 6.4B), the size of the steps would diminish; if a

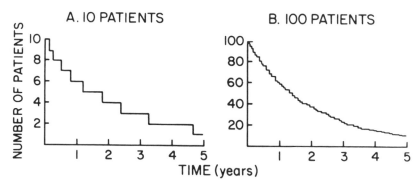

Figure 6.4. Survival of two cohorts, small and large, when all members are observed for the full period of follow-up.

very large number of patients were represented, the figure would approximate a smooth curve. This information could then be used to predict the year-by-year, or even week-by-week, prognosis of similar patients.

Unfortunately, obtaining the information in this way would be quite inefficient for several reasons. Some of the patients would undoubtedly drop out of the study before the end of the follow-up period, perhaps because of another illness, a move to a place where follow-up was impractical, or because of dissatisfaction with the study. These patients would have to be excluded from the cohort, even though considerable effort may have been exerted to gather data on them up to the point at which they dropped out. Also, it would be necessary to wait until all of the cohort's members had reached each point in time before the probability of surviving to that point could be calculated. Because patients ordinarily become available for a study over a period of time, at any point in calendar time there would be a relatively long follow-up for patients who entered the study first, but only brief experience with those who entered recently. The last patient who entered the study would have to reach each year of follow-up before any information on survival to that year would be available.

Survival Curves

In order to make efficient use of all the data, a way of estimating the survival of a cohort over time, called *survival ("life table") analysis,* is used. The purpose of survival analysis is not, as its name implies, only to describe whether patients live or die. Any outcome that is dichotomous and occurs only once during follow-up—for example, time to coronary event, recurrence of cancer, or complete remission—can be described in this way.

Figure 6.5 shows a typical survival curve. On the vertical axis is the probability of surviving, and on the horizontal axis is the period of time following the beginning of observation. Often, the numbers of patients at risk at various points in time are shown to give some idea of the contribution of chance to the observed rates.

With the life table method, the chance of surviving to any point in time is estimated from the cumulative probability of surviving each of the time intervals that preceded it. Time intervals can be made as small as necessary, even days. For the majority of such intervals, no one dies, and the probability of surviving is one. At times, one or more patients die, and the probabilities of surviving at those times are calculated as the ratio of the number of patients surviving to the number at risk of dying at that time. Patients who have already died, dropped out, or have not yet been followed-up to that point are not at risk of dying and so are not used to estimate survival for that time. When patients are lost from the study at any point in time, for any reason, they are called *censored.* The probability of surviving does not change during intervals in which no one dies; so in practice the probability of surviving is recalculated only for times in which there has been a death. Although the probability assigned to any one of the intervals is not very accurate, because of the small number of events

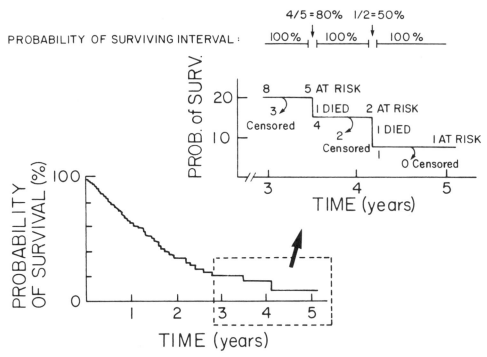

Figure 6.5. A typical survival curve, with detail for one part of the curve.

involved, the overall probability of surviving up to each point in time is remarkably accurate.

A part of the survival curve in Figure 6.5 (from 3 to 5 years after zero time) is presented in detail to illustrate the data used to estimate survival: patients at risk, patients no longer at risk (censored), and patients experiencing outcome events at each point in time.

Interpreting Survival Curves

Several points must be kept in mind when interpreting survival curves. First, the vertical axis represents the probability of surviving for members of a hypothetical cohort, not the percent surviving for an actual cohort. Second, points on a survival curve are the best estimate, for a given set of data, of the probability of survival for members of a cohort. However, the precision of these estimates depends, as do all observations on samples, on the number of observations upon which the estimate is based. One can be more confident that the estimates on the left-hand side of the curve are sound, because more patients are at risk during this time. But at the tail of the curve, on the right, the number of patients upon whom estimates of survival are based often becomes relatively small because deaths, dropouts, and late entrants to the study result in fewer and fewer patients being followed for that length of time. As a result, estimates of survival toward the end of the follow-up period can be strongly affected by what happens to relatively few patients.

In Figure 6.5, the probability of surviving is 8% at 5 years. If at that point the one remaining patient happens to die, the probability of surviving would fall to zero. Clearly this would be a too literal reading of the data. Estimates of survival at the tails of survival curves must, therefore, be interpreted with caution.

Finally, the shape of some survival curves, particularly those in which most patients experience the event of interest, gives the impression that patients die rapidly early on, then reach a plateau at which the risk of dying is considerably less. But this impression is deceptive. As time passes, rates of survival are being applied to a diminishing number of people, and this accounts for the smaller slope of the curve.

Variations on the basic survival curve are found in the medical literature (Fig. 6.6). Often the proportion with, rather than without, the outcome event is indicated on the vertical axis; the curve then sweeps upward and to the right. Other variations increase the amount of information presented with the curve. The number of patients at risk at various points in time can be included; the precision of estimates of survival, which declines with time because fewer and fewer patients are still under observation as time passes, can be identified by confidence intervals (see Chapter 10); and of course survival curves for patients with different characteristics—for example, patients with different prognostic factors or treatments—can be compared in the same figure.

BIAS IN COHORT STUDIES

Regardless of whether cohort studies are used to study risk or prognosis, bias in their conduct can have the effect of creating apparent differences where none actually exist in nature or obscuring differences where they really do exist.

There is the potential for bias in cohort studies, just as for any observations. Bias can be recognized more easily by those who know where in the course of a study it is most likely to occur. They are then in a position to ask important questions that bear on the validity of a study. First, could bias be present under the conditions of the study? Second, is bias actually present in the particular study being considered? Third, are the consequences of bias sufficiently large that they distort the conclusions in a clinically important way? If damage to the study's conclusions is not very great, then the presence of bias may be interesting, but is not responsible for misleading results.

Some of the characteristic locations of bias in cohort research are illustrated in Figure 6.7 and described below.

Assembly Bias

Cohort studies are liable to have a form of selection bias called *assembly*

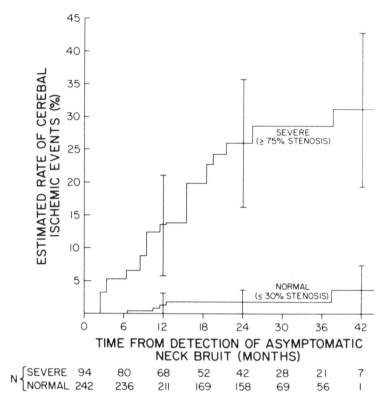

N {
SEVERE 94   80   68   52   42   28   21   7
NORMAL 242   236   211   169   158   69   56   1
}

Figure 6.6. Survival curve showing comparison of two cohorts, number of people at risk, and 95% confidence intervals for observed rates. The cumulative probability of a cerebral ischemic event from time of diagnosis according to the initial degree of carotid stenosis. (Data from Chambers BR, Norris, JW: Outcome in patients with asymptomatic neck bruits. *N Engl J Med* 315:860–865, 1986.)

bias if groups of patients are assembled for study that differ in ways other than the factors under study. These extraneous factors may themselves determine the outcome. If so, observed differences in cohorts at the end of follow-up may simply reflect differences at the beginning and not the particular factors being studied. A comparable term is *susceptibility bias*, which occurs when the groups being compared are not equally susceptible to the outcome of interest, other than for the effects of the factor under study.

Some of the ways in which assembly bias may affect studies of prognosis include differences among cohorts in the extent of disease, the presence of other diseases, the time in the course of disease, and prior treatment. The following illustrates how assembly bias was assessed during a study of patients with Hodgkin's disease.

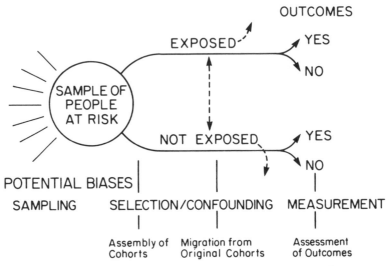

Figure 6.7. Locations of potential bias in cohort studies.

Example—It has been suggested that patients with Hodgkin's disease have a worse prognosis if they have a large mediastinal mass when originally diagnosed. To investigate this assertion, a study was done of 79 patients with Hodgkin's disease, all of whom were initially treated with curative-intent nodal irradiation. Nearly all entered a remission after initial treatment, regardless of the size of the mass. However, patients who initially had large mediastinal masses had a much higher relapse rate (74%) than those with small (27%) or no (19%) mediastinal masses. Could other prognostic factors—particularly, initial stage of disease and symptoms—explain the difference? The authors found that size of mass was related to relapse rate regardless of the stage of disease, and whether or not there were symptoms (Table 6.3). Therefore, size of mediastinal mass was considered an independent prognostic sign. Assembly bias due to staging and symptoms was not present (2).

Migration Bias

Migration bias can occur when patients in one cohort leave their original cohort, either moving to one of the other cohorts under study or dropping out of the study altogether. If these changes take place on a sufficiently large scale, they can affect the validity of conclusions. Migration is another form of selection bias.

In nearly all studies, some members of the original cohort drop out of the study. If these dropouts occur randomly, such that the characteristics of lost subjects in one cohort are on the average similar to those in the other, then no bias would be introduced. This is so whether or not the number of dropouts is similar in the cohorts. But ordinarily the characteristics of lost subjects are not the same in various cohorts. The reasons for

Table 6.3

Analysis of Assembly Bias: The Risk of Recurrence of Hodgkin's Disease According to Size of Mediastinal Mass, Stratified for Stage and Symptoms[a]

	SIZE OF MEDIASTINAL MASS	
	LARGE	SMALL AND NONE
	Recurrence Rate (%)	
Stage		
II	10/14 (71)	6/32 (19)
III	4/4 (100)	7/13 (54)
Symptoms		
No	10/14 (71)	11/41 (27)
Yes	4/4 (100)	2/4 (50)

[a] Data from Lee CKK, Bloomfield CD, Goldman AI, Levitt SH: *Cancer* 46:2403–2409, 1980.

dropping out—death, recovery, side effects of treatment, etc.—are often related to prognosis and may also affect one cohort more than another. As a result, cohorts that were comparable at the outset may become less so as time passes.

Patients may also cross over from one cohort to another during their follow-up. Whenever this occurs, the original reasons for patients falling into one cohort or the other no longer apply. If exchange of patients between cohorts takes place on a large scale, it can diminish the observed difference in risk compared to what might have been observed if the original cohorts had remained intact.

Example—The relationship between exercise and cardiovascular disease was studied by classifying 3975 longshoremen by work activity and observing their rate of fatal heart attacks over a 22-year period. It was recognized that longshoremen originally called active might move to less active jobs, obscuring any relationship that might exist between activity and coronary disease. To deal with this factor, the investigators reclassified the longshoremen's activity each year and looked at risk one year at a time. After adjusting for other risk factors, sedentary workers experienced twice the heart attack rate of the most active group (3).

As the proportion of people in the cohort who are not followed-up increases, the potential for bias increases. It is not difficult to estimate how large this bias could be. All one needs is the number of people in the cohort, the number not accounted for, and the observed outcome rate.

Example—Thompson et al. described the long-term outcomes of gastrogastrostomy (4). A cohort of 123 morbidly obese patients was studied 19–47 months after surgery. Success was defined as having lost more than 30% of excess weight.

Only 103 patients (84%) could be located. In these, the success rate of surgery was 60/103 (58%). To determine the range within which the true success rate must lie, the authors did a best case/worst case analysis. Success rates were calculated assuming that all of the patients lost to follow-up were on the one hand successes (best case) and on the other failures (worst case):

Total cohort = 123
Followed-up = 103
Lost to follow-up = 20

Observed success rate	60/103 = 58%
Best case (all lost patients were successes)	60 + 20/123 = 65%
Worst case (all lost patients were failures)	60/123 = 49%

Thus, the true rate must be between 49 and 65%; probably it is closer to 58%, the observed rate, because patients not followed up are unlikely to be all successes or all failures.

Measurement Bias

Measurement bias is possible if patients in one of the cohorts stand a better chance of having their outcome detected. Obviously some outcomes, such as death, cardiovascular catastrophies, or major cancers, are so obtrusive that they are unlikely to be missed. But for less clear-cut outcomes—the specific cause of death, subclinical disease, side effects, or disability—apparent frequency can be biased by differences in the vigor with which they are sought:

Measurement bias can be minimized in three general ways: One can (a) ensure that those who make the observations are unaware of the group to which patients belong, (b) set careful rules for deciding whether or not an outcome event has occurred (and follow the rules), and (c) apply efforts to discover events equally in all parts of the study.

Example—Chambers and Norris studied the outcome of patients with asymptomatic neck bruits (5). Five hundred asymptomatic patients with cervical bruits were observed for up to 4 years. Patients were classified according to the degree of initial carotid artery stenosis by Doppler ultrasonography. Outcomes were change in degree of carotid stenosis and incidence of cerebral ischemic events.

To avoid biased measurements, the authors estimated carotid stenosis using established, explicit criteria for interpreting Doppler scans and made the readings without knowledge of the auscultatory or previous Doppler findings. Clinical and Doppler assessments were repeated every 6 months, and all noncomplying patients were telephoned to determine whether outcomes had occurred.

This study showed, among other things, that patients with ≥75% carotid stenosis had over a 20% incidence of cerebral ischemic events in 3 years, more than four times the rate of patients with ≤30% stenosis.

Survival Cohorts

In true cohort studies, whether historical or concurrent, patients are assembled at the beginning of the period of time during which they are observed and their course described as it unfolds from that point. True cohort studies should be distinguished from studies of a *survival cohort*, where patients are included in a study because they both have a disease and are currently available—perhaps because they are being seen in a specialized clinic. Another term for such groups of patients is an *available patient cohort*.

In a survival cohort, people are assembled at various times in the course of their disease, rather than at the beginning. Their clinical course is then described by going back in time and seeing how they have fared up to the present (Fig. 6.8).

The experience of survival cohorts are often presented as if they are a description of the course of disease from its inception. However, they are usually a biased view of the course of disease because they include only those patients who are available for study sometime after their disease began. For lethal conditions, the patients in the study are the ones who are fortunate enough to have survived and so are available for observation years later. For diseases that remit, the patients are the ones who are unfortunate enough to have persistent disease. In effect, survival cohorts describe the past history of prevalent cases and not what one would expect over the time following the onset of disease.

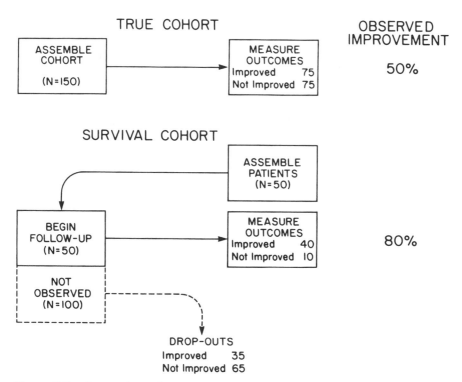

Figure 6.8. Comparison of a true and survival cohort; in the survival cohort, some of the patients present at the beginning are not included in the follow-up.

Reports of survival cohorts are misleading if they are presented as true cohorts. Survival cohorts are relatively prevalent in the medical literature, particularly in the form of "case reports" (to be discussed in Chapter 10).

CONTROLLING FOR SELECTION BIAS

To determine the effect of a factor on prognosis, ideally we would like to compare cohorts with and without the factor, everything else being equal. But in real life "everything else" is usually not equal in cohort studies.

What can be done about this problem? There are several possible ways of *controlling* for differences either during the design or analysis of research (Table 6.4) [a]. For any observational study, if one or more of these strategies has not been applied, the reader should be skeptical. The basic question is: Are the differences in prognosis in the groups related to the particular factor used to distinguish them or to some other factors?

Randomization

The only way to equalize all factors, known and unknown, is to assign the groups randomly, so that each patient has an equal chance of falling into one or the other group. As we mentioned, it is usually not possible to study prognosis in this way. The special situations in which it is possible to allocate exposure randomly, usually to study the effects of treatment on prognosis, will be discussed in Chapter 7.

Restriction

The patients who are enrolled in a study can be restricted to only those possessing a narrow range of characteristics, so that patients do not vary much, one from the other. For example, the effect of age on prognosis after acute myocardial infarction could be studied in white males with uncomplicated anterior myocardial infarctions. One should keep in mind, however, that, although restrictions on entry to a study can certainly produce homogeneous groups, it does so at the expense of generalizability. In the course of excluding potential subjects, cohorts may be selected that are unusual and not representative of most patients with the condition.

Matching

Patients can be matched as they enter the study so that for each patient in one group there are one or more patients in the comparison group with

---

[a] *Control* has several meanings in research:
- A general term for any process—restriction, matching, stratification, adjustment—aimed at removing the effects of extraneous variables while examining the independent effects of one variable
- The nonexposed people in a cohort study (a confusing use of the term)
- The nontreated patients in a clinical trial
- The nondiseased people (noncases) in a case control study

Table 6.4
Methods for Controlling Selection Bias

METHOD	DESCRIPTION	PHASE OF STUDY DESIGN	ANALYSIS
Randomization	Assign patients to groups in a way that gives each patient an equal chance of falling into one or the other group	+	
Restriction	Limit the range of characteristics of patients in the study	+	
Matching	For each patient in one group, select one or more patients with the same characteristics (except for the one under study) for a comparison group	+	
Stratification	Compare rates within subgroups (strata) with otherwise similar probability of the outcome		+
Adjustment Simple	Mathematically adjust crude rates for one or a few characteristics so that equal weight is given to strata of similar risk		+
Multiple	Adjust for differences in a large number of factors related to outcome, using mathematical modeling techniques		+
Best case/ worst case	Describe how different the results could be under the most extreme (or simply very unlikely) conditions of selection bias		+

the same characteristics except for the factor of interest. Often patients are matched for age and sex, because these factors are strongly related to the prognosis of many diseases. But matching for other factors may be called for as well, such as stage or severity of disease, rate of progression, and prior treatments. An example of matching in a cohort study of sickle cell trait was presented in the discussion of observational studies in Chapter 5.

Although matching is commonly used and can be very useful, it controls for bias only for those factors involved in the match. Also, it is usually not possible to match for more than a few factors, because of practical difficulties in finding patients who meet all the matching criteria. Moreover, if categories for matching are relatively crude, there may be room for substantial differences between matched groups. For example, if a study of risk for Down's syndrome were conducted in which there was matching for maternal age within 10 years, there could be a nearly 10-fold difference in frequency related to age if most of the women in one group were 30 and most in the other 39. Also, once one restricts or matches on a variable, its effects on outcomes can no longer be evaluated in the study.

Stratification

After data are collected, they can be analyzed and results presented according to subgroups of patients, or *strata*, of similar characteristics.

Example—Let us suppose we want to compare the operative mortality rates for coronary bypass surgery at Hospitals A and B. Overall, Hospital A noted 48 deaths in 1200 bypass operations (4%) and Hospital B experienced 64 deaths in 2400 operations (2.6%).

The crude rates suggest that hospital B is superior. Or do they? Perhaps patients in the two hospitals were not otherwise of comparable prognosis. On the basis of age, myocardial function, extent of occlusive disease, and other characteristics, the patients can be divided into subgroups based on preoperative risk (Table 6.5); then the operative mortality rates within each category or stratum of risk can be compared.

Table 6.5 shows that, when patients are divided by preoperative risk, the operative mortality rates in each risk stratum are identical in two hospitals: 6% in high risk patients, 4% in medium risk patients, and 0.67% in low risk patients. The obvious source of the misleading impression created by examining only the crude rates is the important differences in the risk characteristics of the patients treated at the two hospitals: 42% of A's patients and only 17% of B's patients were high risk.

Stratification is one of the most common and most revealing ways of examining for bias, particularly confounding bias.

Standardization

Two rates can be compared without bias if they are adjusted so as to equalize the weight given to another factor that could be related to outcome. This process, called *standardization* (or *adjustment*), shows what the overall rate would be if strata-specific rates were applied to a population made up

Table 6.5
Example of Stratification: Death Rates after Coronary Bypass Surgery in Two Hospitals, Stratified by Preoperative Risk[a]

PREOPERATIVE RISK	HOSPITAL A			HOSPITAL B		
	PATIENTS	DEATHS	RATE	PATIENTS	DEATHS	RATE
			(%)			(%)
High	500	30	6	400	24	6
Medium	400	16	4	800	32	4
Low	300	2	0.67	1200	8	0.67
Total	1200	48	4	2400	64	2.6

[a] Fictitious data.

of similar proportions of people in each stratum. In the previous example, the high risk mortality rate of 6% receives a weight of 500/1200 in Hospital A and a much lower weight of 400/2400 in Hospital B, and so on such that the crude rate for Hospital A equals $(500/1200 \times 0.06) + (400/1200 \times 0.04) + (300/1200 \times 0.0067)$ or 0.04 and the crude rate for Hospital B equals $(400/2400 \times 0.06) + (800/2400 \times 0.04) + (1200/2400 \times 0.0067)$ or 0.026.

If equal weights are used, let us say 1/3 (but they could be based on one or the other hospital or any reference population), then the standardized rate for Hospital A equals $(1/3 \times 0.06) + (1/3 \times 0.04) + (1/3 \times 0.0067)$ or 0.036, which is exactly the same as the standardized rate for Hospital B. The consequence of giving equal weight to strata in each group is to remove totally the apparent excess risk of Hospital A.

The difference between the crude operative mortality rates in the two hospitals results from the bias introduced by the differences in patients' preoperative risk. We are only interested in differences attributable to the hospitals and their surgeons, not to the patients per se. The difference in the crude mortality rates is confounded by the differences in patients, whereas the absence of a difference in the standardized incidence rates is unbiased, unconfounded, or controlled.

Multivariable Adjustment

In most clinical situations, many factors act together to produce effects. The associations among these variables are complex: They may be related to each other, as well as to the outcome of interest; the effect of one might be modified by the presence of others; and the joint effects of two or more might be greater than the sum of their individual effects.

Multivariable analysis is a method for simultaneously considering the effects of many variables. It is done by developing a mathematical expression (*model*) based on the data and some assumptions, relating independent variables to outcome. Computer programs for performing multivariable analysis are widely available. Methods commonly used in clinical research include multiple linear and logistic regression.

In general, multivariable analysis is used to adjust (control) simultaneously for the effects of many variables in order to determine the independent effects of one. Also, the method can select from a large set of variables a smaller subset that independently and significantly contributes to the overall variation in outcome and can arrange variables in order of the strength of their contribution.

Multivariable analysis is the only feasible way to deal with many variables at one time. Simpler methods, such as stratification or matching, can only consider a few variables at a time and then only by sacrificing statistical power. Yet, multivariable analysis has disadvantages. The internal workings of the method are a "black box" to most clinicians and many researchers. The models are based on assumptions that may not be met by the data. Also, it is often uncertain how the order in which variables are entered in the model, multiple comparisons, statistical power, and associations among variables affect the results.

Sensitivity Analysis

When data on important prognostic factors are not available, it is possible to estimate the potential effects on the study by assuming various degrees of maldistribution of the factors between the groups being compared and seeing how that would affect the results. The general term for this process is *sensitivity analysis.* [b] A special case, when one compares results assuming the best and worst possible maldistribution of a prognostic variable, is called a *best case/worst case analysis.*

Assuming the worst is a particularly stringent test of how a factor might affect the conclusions of a study. A less conservative approach is to assume that the factor is distributed between the groups in an unlikely way.

Example—The University Group Diabetes Program (UGDP) study of treatment for mild diabetes found that patients given tolbutamide experienced a greater risk of dying from cardiovascular disease than those given insulin or diet alone. The results were criticized because data on smoking (which is associated with cardiovascular death) were not collected and not taken into account in the analysis. It was suggested that, if cigarette smokers were unequally distributed among the groups, such that there were more smokers among those receiving tolbutamide than in the other groups, then the difference in death rates might be related to smoking, not tolbutamide. However, Cornfield has pointed out that even if cigarette smokers in the tolbutamide group exceeded those in the control group by 20%, a situation that would have been extremely unlikely by chance (1/50,000), an increased risk in the tolbutamide group would have persisted. Thus, bias in the distribution of smokers could not have accounted for the observed differences (6).

Overall Strategy

All of these ways of dealing with extraneous differences between groups other than by randomization have a limitation. They are effective against only those factors that are known to be related to outcome and are singled out for consideration. They do not deal with prognostic factors that are not known at the time of the study or are known but not taken into account.

Ordinarily, one does not rely on only one or another method of controlling for bias; one uses several methods together, layered one on another. Thus, in a study of whether the presence of ventricular premature contractions decreases survival in the years following acute myocardial infarction, one might (a) restrict the study to patients who are not very old or young

---

[b] A sensitivity analysis of the effects of incomplete follow-up has been presented in this chapter. Sensitivity analysis can also be used to assess the potential effects of inaccuracies in the data used in decision analysis.

and do not have unusual causes (for example, mycotic aneurysm) for their infarction; (b) match for age, a factor strongly related to prognosis but extraneous to the main question; (c) examine the results separately for strata of differing clinical severity (for example, the presence or absence of congestive heart failure or other diseases, such as chronic obstructive pulmonary disease); and (d) finally, adjust the crude results for the effects of all the variables other than the arrhythmia, taken together, that might be related to prognosis.

SUMMARY

Prognosis is a description of the course of disease from its onset. Compared to risk, prognostic events are relatively frequent and often can be estimated by personal clinical experience. However, cases of disease ordinarily seen in medical centers and reported in the medical literature are often biased samples of all cases and tend to overestimate severity.

Prognosis is best described by the probability of having experienced an outcome event at any time in the course of disease. In principle, this can be done by observing a cohort until all who will experience the outcome of interest have done so. However, because this approach is inefficient, another method, called life table analysis, is often used. The onset of events over time is estimated by accumulating the rates for all patients at risk during the preceding time intervals.

As for any observations on cohorts, studies comparing prognosis can be biased if differences arise because of the way cohorts are assembled, whether or not patients remain in their initial cohorts, and whether outcome is assessed equally. A variety of strategies are available to deal with such differences as might arise, so as to allow fair (unbiased) comparisons. They should be found whenever comparisons are made.

REFERENCES

1. Percy AK, Nobrega FT, Okazaki H, Glattre E, Kurland LT: Multiple sclerosis in Rochester, Minn. A 60-year appraisal. *Arch Neurol* 25:105–111, 1971.
2. Lee CKK, Bloomfield CD, Goldman AI, Levitt SH: Prognostic significance of mediastinal involvement in Hodgkin's disease treated with curative radiotherapy. *Cancer* 42:2403–2409, 1980.
3. Brand RJ, Paffenbarger RS, Sholtz RI, Kampert JB: Work activity and fatal heart attack studied by multiple logistic risk analysis. *Am J Epidemiol* 110:52–62, 1979.
4. Thompson KS, Fletcher SW, O'Malley MS, Buckwalter JA: Long-term outcomes of morbidly obese patients treated with gastrogastrostomy. *J Gen Intern Med* 1:85–89, 1986.
5. Chambers BR, Norris JW: Outcome in patients with asymptomatic neck bruits. *N Engl J Med* 315:860–865, 1986.
6. Cornfield J: The University Group Diabetes Program. A further statistical analysis of the mortality findings. *JAMA* 217:1676–1687, 1971.

SUGGESTED READINGS

Colton T: Longitudinal studies and use of the life table. In *Statistics in Medicine.* Boston, Little, Brown and Co, 1974.

Feinstein AR: *Clinical Biostatistics.* St. Louis, CV Mosby, 1977.

Feinstein AR, Sosin DM, Wells CK: The Will Rogers phenomenon—Stage migration and new diagnostic techniques as a source of misleading statistics for survival in cancer. *N Engl J Med* 312:1604–1608, 1985.

Feinstein AR: *Clinical Epidemiology. The Architecture of Clinical Research.* Philadelphia, WB Saunders, 1985.

Horwitz RI: The experimental paradigm and observational studies of cause-effect relationships in clinical medicine. *J. Chron Dis* 40:91–99, 1987.

Motulsky AG: Biased ascertainment and the natural history of diseases. *N Engl J Med* 298:1196–1197, 1978.

Murphy EA: Survivorship functions. In *Probability in Medicine.* Baltimore, Johns Hopkins University Press, 1979.

Peto R, Pike MC, Armitage P, Breslow NE, Cox DR, Howard SV, Mantel N, McPherson K, Peto J, Smith PG: Design and analysis of randomized clinical trials requiring prolonged observation of each patient. II. Analysis and examples. *Br J Cancer* 35:1–39, 1977.

Rothman KJ: *Modern Epidemiology.* Boston, Little, Brown and Co, 1986.

Wasson JH, Sox HC, Neff RK, Goldman L: Clinical prediction rules. Applications and methodological standards. *N Engl J Med* 313:793–799, 1985.

Weiss NS: *Clinical Epidemiology. The Study of the Outcomes of Illness.* New York, Oxford University Press, 1986.

APPENDIX 6.1. MAIN QUESTIONS FOR DETERMINING THE VALIDITY OF STUDIES OF INCIDENCE (NOT INVOLVING COMPARISONS)[a]

1. Is there a defined *cohort* with all members:
   • *Described* (characteristics and inclusion/exclusion criteria)?
   • *Entered at the beginning of follow-up?*
   • *At risk* for developing the outcome?
   • At similar *zero time* (point in the course of disease)?
2. *Is the time period of follow-up described for each patient and is it:*
   • *Complete* (or if there are dropouts, are they few and/or is there an unbiased sample of those that remain)?
   • *Long enough* for outcome events to occur?
3. *Are criteria for outcome events* described?

---

[a] These questions are not meant to be all-inclusive nor to replace independent, critical thinking. They are a rough guideline, including only the most basic elements of sound study.

chapter 7

Treatment

Once the nature of a patient's illness has been established and its expected course predicted, the next question is: What can be done about it? Is there a treatment that improves the outcome of disease? This chapter describes ways of deciding whether a well-intentioned treatment does in fact do more good than harm.

IDEAS AND EVIDENCE

Ideas about what might be useful treatment arise from virtually any activity within medicine.

Some therapeutic hypotheses are suggested by the mechanisms of disease at the cellular or molecular level. The combination of antibiotics, trimethoprim-sulfamethoxazole, resulted from research on folic acid metabolism. Such drugs as cimetidine, corticosteroids, L-dopa, H_2 and β-blockers, and many antimetabolites were discovered through basic biomedical research.

Other hypotheses about the value of treatment have come from astute observations by clinicians. Two recent examples are the discovery that patients with Parkinson's disease, given amantadine to prevent influenza, show improvement in their neurologic status, and reports that colchicine, given for gout, reduces the frequency of attacks of familial Mediterranean fever. The value of these treatments was not predicted by an understanding of the mechanism of these diseases, and the ways in which these drugs work are not yet understood.

Ideas about treatment also come from epidemiologic studies of populations. Burkitt observed that colonic diseases are relatively infrequent in African countries, where diet is high in fiber, compared to developed countries where intake of dietary fiber is low. This observation has led to efforts to prevent bowel diseases—irritable bowel syndrome, diverticulitis, appendicitis, and colorectal cancer—with high fiber diets.

Testing Ideas

Some treatments are so powerful that their value is self-evident even without formal testing. We do not have reservations about the value of penicillin for pneumonia, surgery for appendicitis, or thyroid hormone replacement for hypothyroidism. Clinical experience has been sufficient.

Usually, however, the effects of treatment are considerably less dramatic. It is then necessary to put ideas about treatments to a formal test, because a variety of conditions—coincidence, faulty comparisons, spontaneous changes in the course of disease, wishful thinking, etc.—can obscure the true relationship between treatment and effect. As Lewis Thomas put it, "Hunches and intuitive impressions are essential for getting the work started, but it is only through the quality of the numbers at the end that the truth can be told" (1).

For some clinical problems knowledge of disease mechanisms, based on work with laboratory models or physiologic studies in humans, has become so extensive that it is tempting to predict effects in humans without formal testing. Relying solely on our current understanding of mechanisms, without testing out ideas on intact humans, however, can lead to unpleasant surprises.

Example—Many strokes are caused by cerebral infarction in the area distal to an obstructed segment of the internal carotid artery. It should be possible to prevent the manifestations of disease from progressing, in people with these lesions, by bypassing the diseased segment so that blood can flow to the threatened area normally. It is technically feasible to anastamose the superficial temporal artery to the internal carotid distal to an obstruction. Because its value seemed self-evident on physiologic grounds, and because of the documented success of an analogous procedure, coronary artery bypass surgery, the procedure became widely used.

The EC/IC Bypass Study Group conducted a randomized controlled trial of temporal artery bypass surgery (2). Patients with cerebral ischemia and an obstructed internal carotid artery were randomly allocated to surgical versus medical treatment. The operation was a technical success; 96% of anastomoses were patent just after surgery. Yet, the surgery did not help the patients. Mortality and stroke rates after 5 years were nearly identical in the surgically and medically treated patients, but deaths occurred earlier in the surgically treated patients.

This study illustrates how treatments that make good sense, based on what we know about the mechanisms of disease, may be found ineffective in human terms when put to a rigorous test.

Therefore, it is almost always necessary to test therapeutic hypotheses by means of clinical research, in which data are collected on the clinical course of patients who have actually experienced the treatment. As one author put it, treatments should be given "not because they ought to work, but because they do work" (3).

STUDIES OF TREATMENT EFFECTS

Treatment is usually considered to be what physicians prescribe for patients with established disease: surgery, drugs, exercise, diet, etc. But it should be evident that there are a great many other ways of intervening to improve health. Among these are efforts to prevent disease (discussed in the next chapter) as well as interventions in communities, rather than individuals, or changes in the organization and financing of health care. Regardless of the nature of a well-intentioned intervention, the principles by which it is judged superior to its alternatives are the same.

Studies of treatment are a special case of studies of prognosis in general, where the particular factor of interest is a therapeutic intervention. Therefore, what has been said about cohort studies (Chapters 5 and 6) applies to studies of treatment as well. Observational studies are in fact one way of assessing treatment. However, because systematic differences in treatment groups occur frequently when they are compared by means of observational studies, it is preferable to impose more order on the comparison.

Clinical Trials

Clinical trials are a special kind of cohort study in which the conditions of study—selection of treatment groups, nature of interventions, management during follow-up, etc.—are specified by the investigator for the purpose of making unbiased comparisons. Clinical trials, thus, are more highly controlled and managed than are cohort studies. The investigators are, in effect, conducting an experiment, analogous to those done in the laboratory. They have taken it upon themselves (with their patients' permission) to isolate for study the unique contribution of one factor by holding constant, as much as possible, all other determinants of the outcome. Hence, other names for clinical trials are *intervention* or *experimental* studies.

The structure of a clinical trial, in a simplified form, is shown in Figure 7.1. The patients to be studied are first selected from a larger number of patients with the condition of interest. They are then divided into two groups of comparable prognosis. One group, called the *experimental* or treated group, is exposed to some intervention that is believed to be helpful. The other group, called a *control* or comparison group, is treated the same in all ways except that its members are not exposed to the intervention. The clinical course of both groups is then observed, and any differences in outcome are attributed to the intervention.

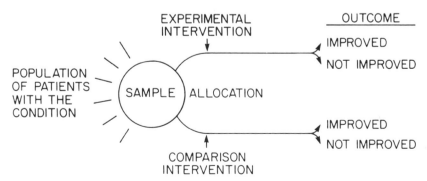

Figure 7.1.   The structure of a clinical trial.

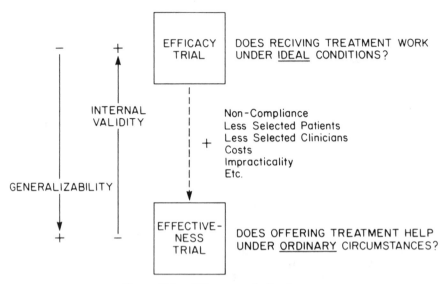

Figure 7.2. Efficacy and effectiveness.

The main reason for structuring clinical trials in this way is to avoid bias, or systematic error, when comparing the respective value of the two or more kinds of managements. The validity of clinical trials depends on how well they result in an equal distribution of all determinants of prognosis, other than the one being tested, in treated and control patients.

In the following discussion, we will describe the design and interpretation of clinical trials. We will then place clinical trials in context with other studies of clinical interventions.

Efficacy, Effectiveness, and Compliance

A trial's results are judged in reference to two broad questions: Can the treatment work under ideal circumstances? Does it work in ordinary settings? The words "efficacy" and "effectiveness" have been applied to these concepts (Fig. 7.2).[a]

The question of whether a treatment can work is one of *efficacy*. An *efficacious* treatment is one that does more good than harm among those who receive it. Efficacy is established by restricting patients in a study to those who will cooperate fully with medical advice.

In contrast, a treatment is *effective* if it does more good than harm in those to whom it is offered. Effectiveness is established by offering a treatment or program to patients and allowing them to accept or reject it as they might ordinarily do. Only a small proportion of clinical trials set

[a] The distinction between efficacy and effectiveness is not found in the dictionary. These words have been given specific meanings in order to express important concepts in medical care.

out to answer questions of effectiveness. This is in part because of the risk that the result will be inconclusive: If a treatment is found to be ineffective, it may be due to lack of efficacy, lack of patient acceptance, or both.

Compliance is the extent to which patients follow medical advice. Some have preferred the term "adherence," because it has a less dictatorial connotation. Compliance intervenes between an efficacious treatment and an effective one.

Although noncompliance suggests a kind of willful neglect of good advice, other factors also contribute. Patients may misunderstand which drugs and doses are intended, run out of prescription medications, confuse various (generic) preparations of the same drug, or have no money or insurance to pay for drugs. Taken together, these may limit the usefulness of treatments that have been shown to be efficacious under specially favorable conditions.

Compliance is particularly important in medical care outside the hospital. In the hospital, many factors act to constrain patients' personal behavior and render them compliant. Hospitalized patients are generally sicker and more frightened. They are in strange surroundings, dependent on the skill and attention of the staff for everything—even their life. What is more, doctors, nurses, and pharmacists have developed a well-organized system for ensuring that patients receive what is ordered for them. As a result, clinical experience and a medical literature developed on the wards may underestimate the importance of compliance outside the hospital, where most patients and doctors are and where patients have much greater freedom of choice.

Sampling

The kinds of patients that are included in a trial determine the extent to which conclusions can be generalized to other patients. Of the many reasons why patients with the condition of interest may not be part of a trial, three account for most of the losses: They do not meet specific inclusion/exclusion criteria, they refuse to participate, or they are considered unlikely to cooperate with treatment once they have entered the trial.

The first, inclusion/exclusion criteria, is intended to restrict the heterogeneity of patients in the trial and to improve the chances of patients completing the assigned treatment. Common exclusion criteria are atypical disease, the presence of other diseases, an unusually poor prognosis (which may cause patients to drop out of the assigned treatment group), and contraindications to one of the treatments. As heterogeneity is restricted in this way, the internal validity of the study is improved; there is less opportunity for variation in outcome that is not related to treatment in the groups being compared. But exclusions come at the price of diminished generalizability because characteristics that exclude patients occur commonly among patients ordinarily seen in clinical practice.

Second, patients can refuse to participate in a trial. They may not want a particular type of treatment or to have their medical care decided by someone other than their own physician. Patients who refuse to participate are likely to be systematically different—in socioeconomic class, severity of disease, other health-related problems, etc.—from those who agree to enter the trial.

Third, patients who are thought to be unreliable, so that they may not follow the groundrules of the trial, are usually not enrolled in the first place. This avoids wasted effort and the reduction in internal validity that would occur if patients moved in and out of treatment groups or out of the trial altogether.

For these reasons, patients in clinical trials are usually a highly selected, biased sample of all patients with the condition of interest. Because of the high degree of selection in trials, it often requires considerable faith to generalize the results of clinical trials to ordinary practice settings.

Figure 7.3 shows how patients were selected for a trial of surgery versus medical therapy for coronary artery disease (4). A total of 16,626 patients at 11 sites were considered for entry into the trial if they had undergone coronary angiography because of suspected coronary artery disease. In the end, only 780 of the 16,626 patients (4.7%) entered the trial.

THE INTERVENTION

The intervention itself can be described in relation to four general characteristics.

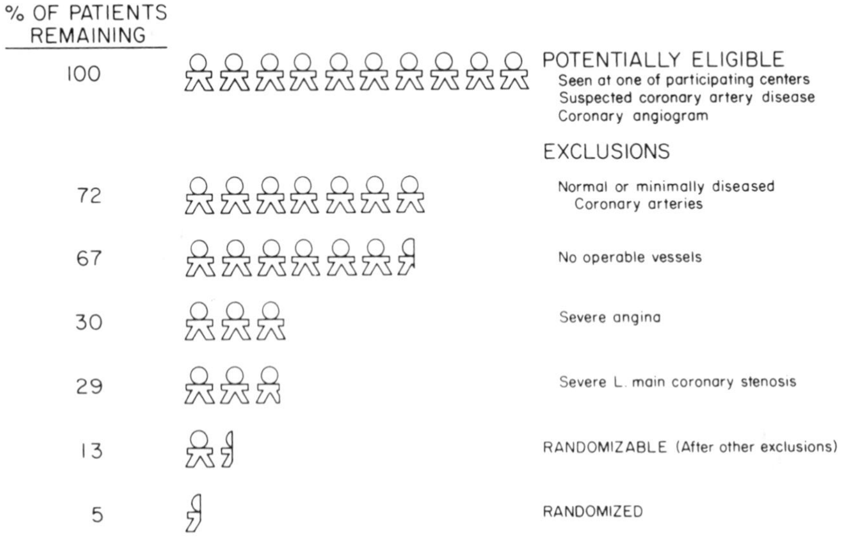

Figure 7.3. Sampling for a clinical trial: the Coronary Artery Surgery Study (CASS). (Data from CASS Principal Investigators and their Associates: Coronary Artery Surgery Study (CASS): a randomized trial of coronary artery bypass surgery. Survival data. *Circulation* 68:939–950, 1983.)

Generalizability

Is the intervention in question one that is likely to be implemented in usual clinical practice? In an effort to standardize therapy so as to have it easily described and reproducible in other settings, some investigators end up studying treatments that are so unlike those ordinarily used that the results of the trial are not useful.

Complexity

Single, highly specific interventions make for tidy science, because they can be described precisely and applied in a reproducible way. However, clinicians regularly make choices among alternative treatments that involve many elements. Examples include whether to manage a patient with pulmonary edema in an intensive care unit or on the ward and whether to request chest physiotherapy for patients with respiratory failure or speech rehabilitation for patients with aphasia. All these interventions are amenable to careful evaluation, as long as their essence can be communicated and reproduced in other settings.

Example—Although most patients with acute myocardial infarction (AMI) are treated in coronary care units (CCUs), evidence that this is the best policy is not conclusive. A study was done in England to determine if there is a difference in early mortality from AMI among patients treated in CCUs, compared to those treated at home.

It was possible to assign 264 of 369 patients (76%) suspected of having AMI to home or hospital care. All patients were visited in their homes, shortly after the onset of symptoms, and a preliminary diagnosis was made. Patients in one group were sent to a regional hospital, where they were admitted to a CCU and cared for in the usual way. The other patients remained at home and were cared for by their general practitioner.

There was no significant difference in 6-week mortality between the home group (13%) and the hospital group (11%). Although the specific components of care in the home and hospital were neither determined by the investigators nor described in detail, it was apparent that these interventions represented care that might ordinarily be given under such circumstances. Thus, the usual policy of admitting all patients to CCUs was not supported, at least for the majority of patients in a community who were suspected of having an AMI (5).

Strength

Is the intervention in question sufficiently different from alternative managements that it is reasonable to expect that outcome will be affected? Some diseases can be reversed by treating a single, dominant cause, e.g., thyroid ablation for hyperthyroidism. But most diseases are determined by a combination of factors acting in concert. Interventions that change only one of them, and only a small amount, cannot be expected to show strong treatment effects. If the conclusion of a trial evaluating such interventions is that a new treatment is not effective, it comes as no surprise.

Obsolescence

Is it possible that changes in patient management have rendered the results of a trial obsolete, even before they become available? Physicians have a tendency to adopt new ways of managing disease, particularly if they make physiologic sense, before they have been rigorously evaluated. Trials often take years to complete, and conventional management may have changed substantially while a trial of one component of management is being conducted. Consequently, when the results of a trial become available they are at risk of being considered irrelevant to current medical practice. But without these trials, clinicians' information base would be like the flight plan for a pilot, somewhere over the ocean, who reported to his passengers, "We're lost—but we're making record time!"

COMPARISON GROUPS

Obviously the value of a treatment can only be judged by comparing its results to those of some alternative course of action. The question is not whether a point of comparison is used, but how appropriate it is. In clinical trials, comparison groups can be identified with all degrees of formality—from innuendo to carefully selected, highly comparable controls.

Uncontrolled Trials

Trials are called *uncontrolled* if they specifically describe the course of disease only in a single group of patients who have been exposed to a particular intervention of interest.

What is wrong with assessing the effects of treatment by comparing clinical courses in patients before and after treatment? The results can be misleading for several reasons.

- **Unpredictable Outcome**
When the clinical course of a disease is quite predictable, a separate control group is less important. We know that subacute bacterial endocarditis left untreated invariably leads to death, that most patients with hypothyroidism will only get worse instead of better without exogenous thyroid hormone, and that bowel infarction will not improve without surgery.

However, most therapeutic decisions do not involve diseases with such predictable outcomes. In situations where the clinical course is extremely variable for a given patient and from one patient to another, assessing treatment effects by observing changes in the course of disease after treatment is unreliable.

Many severe diseases that are not self-limited may nevertheless undergo spontaneous remissions in activity that can be misinterpreted as treatment effects. Figure 7.4 shows the clinical course, over a 10-year period, of a patient with systemic lupus erythematosus. Although powerful treatments were not given (because none was available during most of the years

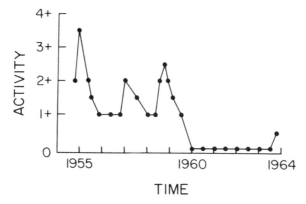

TIME

Figure 7.4. The unpredictable course of disease: the natural history of systemic lupus erythematosus in a patient observed before the advent of immunosuppressive drugs. (Redrawn from Ropes M: *Systemic Lupus Erythematosus.* Cambridge, Harvard University Press, 1976.)

shown), the disease passed through dramatic periods of exacerbation, followed by prolonged remissions. Of course, exacerbations, such as those illustrated, are alarming to both patients and doctors, so there is often a feeling that something must be done at these times. If treatment were begun at the peak of activity, improvement would have followed. Without any better comparison than the previous activity of the disease, the treatment would have received credit for the improvement.

- **Hawthorne Effect**
   A great deal of special attention is directed toward patients in clinical trials, and they are well aware of it. Patients may improve because of this attention and not because of the treatment itself.
   The *Hawthorne effect* is the tendency for people to change their behavior because they are the target of special interest and attention in a study, regardless of the specific nature of the intervention they might be receiving.[b] It is not clear what all the reasons for this changed behavior are. But patients are anxious to please their doctors and make them feel successful. Also, patients who volunteer for trials want to do their part to see that "good" results are obtained.
   There is no way of separating out Hawthorne from treatment effects in uncontrolled trials. But if there are control patients who receive the same attention as the treated ones, then the Hawthorne effect cancels out in the comparison.

---

[b] The term "Hawthorne effect" stems from studies done in the 1920s at the Hawthorne Works of the Western Electric Company in Chicago. Workers exposed to varying levels of illumination intensity increased their work output whether the intensity had increased, decreased, or remained the same. It was apparent that characteristics of the study situation other than illumination were responsible for the observed changes. This work is summarized in Roethlisberger FJ, Dickson WJ, Wright HA: *Management and the Worker.* Cambridge, MA, 1946.

- **Regression to the Mean**

Treatments are often tried because a manifestation of disease is extreme or unusual—for example, a particularly high blood pressure or fever. In this situation, subsequent measurements are likely to show improvement for purely statistical reasons.

As discussed in Chapter 2, patients selected because they represent an extreme value in a distribution are likely, on the average, to have lower values for later measurements. If those patients are treated after first being found abnormal, and the effects of treatment assessed by subsequent measurements, improvement could be expected even if treatment were ineffective. Regression to the mean is therefore another reason why using patients as their own controls can be misleading.

- **Predictable Improvement**

If the usual course of a disease is to improve, then therapeutic efforts may coincide with improvement but not cause it. For many acute, self-limited diseases—upper respiratory infections or gastroenteritis—patients tend to seek care when the symptoms are at their worst. They often begin to recover after seeing the doctor because of the natural course of events regardless of what was done.

Comparisons across Time and Place

Control patients can be chosen from a time and place different from the experimental patients. For example, we may compare the prognosis of recent patients, treated with current medications, to experience with past patients who were treated when those medications were not available. Similarly, we may compare the results of surgery in one hospital to results in another where a different procedure is used. This approach is convenient. The problem is that time and place are almost always strongly related to prognosis. Clinical trials that attempt to make fair comparisons between groups of patients arising in different eras, or in different settings, have a particularly difficult task.

Time

The results of current treatment are sometimes compared to experience with similar patients in the past—*historical* or *nonconcurrent controls.* Although it may be done well, this design has many pitfalls. Methods of diagnosis and treatment change with time, and with them the average prognosis. It has been shown that trials with historical controls can be misleading.

Example—Sacks et al. reviewed clinical trials of six therapies to see if trials with concurrent, as compared to historical, controls produced different results (6). They studied 50 randomized trials and 56 studies with historical controls. Seventy-nine percent of trials with historical controls found the experimental treatment to be better, but only 20% of trials with a concurrent, randomized control group found treatment to be better. Differences between the two kinds of trials occurred mainly because the control patients in the historical trials did worse. Adjustment for prognostic factors, when possible, did not change the results; that is, the differences were due to general improvements in therapy or to selection of less ill patients.

Therefore, if concurrent, randomized controlled trials are taken as a standard of validity it seems that published historical trials are biased in favor of the experimental treatment and that the bias cannot be overcome by adjusting for known prognostic variables.

If historical controls are used, the shorter the period of time between selection of treated and control groups and the less other aspects of medical care have changed during the interval, the safer the comparison. Thus, some oncology centers study a succession of chemotherapeutic regimens by comparing results of the newest regimen to those of the immediately preceding one, often given as recently as the previous year. In general, however, choosing *concurrent controls* (i.e., patients treated during the same period of time) avoids a potential source of bias.

Place

Experience in other settings, using different treatments, can serve as a standard of comparison. However, it is preferable to choose both treated and control patients from the same setting because a variety of factors— referral patterns, organization and skill of staff, etc.—often result in very different prognoses in different settings, independently of the treatment under study.

Example—In a study of anticoagulants and acute myocardial infarction, in 22 hospitals the 21-day mortality among patients given anticoagulants ranged from 0–40% (Fig. 7.5). Even if consideration were limited only to those hospitals where enough patients were studied to give a reasonably reliable estimate of death rate, the range was 5.3–21.0%. Differences in mortality rates among hospitals were larger than differences attributed to treatment. If the value of anticoagulants had been studied by comparing death rates in a hospital using anticoagulants to another that did not, and the hospitals happened to be ones with quite different death rates in any case, a misleading conclusion would have resulted (7).

Which Comparison Treatment?

A new treatment is either better, the same, or worse compared to some implied standard. Without defining the control (comparison) treatment, reports of the efficacy of experimental treatments cannot be interpreted.

Results among patients receiving an experimental treatment can be measured against one or more of several kinds of comparison groups:

• **No Intervention**
Do patients receiving the experimental treatment end up better than before treatment? Here, the comparison is to the baseline state. Because of regression to the mean, diseases that wax and wane often improve regardless of treatment if they are identified at a particularly severe phase in their

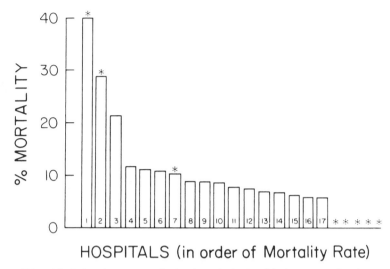

HOSPITALS (in order of Mortality Rate)

Figure 7.5. Variation in prognosis by hospital: the 21-day mortality from acute myocardial infarction for patients treated with anticoagulants in 22 hospitals. Hospitals designated by an asterisk had less than 10 patients. (Data from Modan B, Shani M, Schor S, Modan M: Reduction of hospital mortality from acute myocardial infarction by anticoagulant therapy. *N Engl J Med* 292:1359–1362, 1975.)

course. On the other hand, diseases with a uniformly downhill course may only stabilize with an effective treatment.

• **Observation**

Do treated patients do better than other patients who are simply observed? As described earlier, people have a tendency to change their behavior when they are the target of special interest and attention in a study, regardless of the specific nature of the intervention they may be receiving.

• **Placebo Treatment**

Do treated patients do better than similar patients given a placebo? A *placebo* is an intervention that is intended to be indistinguishable from the active treatment—in physical appearance, color, taste, odor, etc.—but does not have a specific, known mechanism of action. Sugar pills and saline injections are examples of placebos. It has been shown that placebos, given with conviction, relieve severe, unpleasant symptoms, such as postoperative pain, nausea, or itching, of about one-third of patients, a phenomenon called the *placebo effect*.

Example—Patients with chronic severe itching were entered in a trial of antipruritic drugs. During each of 3 weeks, 46 patients received in random order either cyproheptadine HCl (Periactin), trimeprazine tartrate (Temaril), or placebo. There was a 1-week rest period, randomly introduced into the sequence, in which no pills were given. Results were assessed without knowledge of medication and expressed as "itching scores" (Table 7.1). The two active drugs and placebo were all similarly effective. Both drugs and placebo gave much better results than when nothing at all was given (8).

Placebo effects have different meaning for researchers and clinicians. Researchers are more likely to be interested in establishing specific effects—ones that are consistent with current theories about the causes of disease. They consider the placebo effect the baseline against which to measure specific effects.

On the other hand, clinicians should understand that all of their interventions have both specific and nonspecific effects (Fig. 7.6). They should welcome the placebo effect and attempt to maximize it, or any other way of helping patients. What is most important is the total effect of the intervention beyond what would have otherwise occurred in the course of disease without treatment. However, it is also useful to know what part of the total effect is specific and what is nonspecific so as to avoid dangerous, uncomfortable, or costly interventions when relatively little of their effect can be attributed to their specific actions.

Table 7.1
The Placebo Effect: Control of Chronic Itching by Two "Active Drugs" and a Placebo, Compared to No Treatment (36 Patients)[a]

DRUG	ITCHING SCORE[b]
Cyproheptadine HCl	28
Trimeprazine tartrate	35
Placebo	30
Nothing	50

[a] Data from Fischer RW: *JAMA* 203:418–419, 1968.
[b] The higher the score, the more the itching.

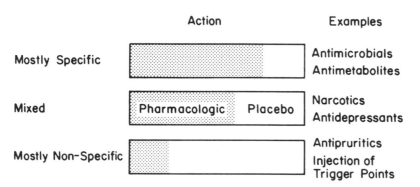

Figure 7.6.   The effects of most drugs are partly attributable to the placebo effect. (Redrawn from Fletcher RH: The clinical importance of placebo effects. *Fam Med Rev* 1:40–48, 1983.)

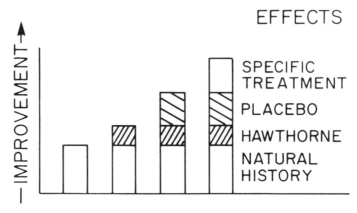

Figure 7.7.   Total effects of treatment are the sum of spontaneous improvement, nonspecific responses, and the effects of specific treatments.

- **Usual Treatment**

  Do patients given the experimental treatment do better than those receiving the usual treatment? This is the only meaningful (and ethical) question if the usual treatment is already known to be efficacious.

  The cumulative effects of these various sources of improvement are diagrammed in Figure 7.7.

ALLOCATING TREATMENT

If it can be accepted that a concurrent control group is preferable, what is the most effective way of assigning patients to receive a new treatment or serve as controls?

Nonrandom Allocation

One way to allocate patients to treated and control groups is to have the physicians in charge of the patients' care decide. When this is done, the study has all the advantages and disadvantages of cohort studies.

Studies of treated cohorts take advantage of the fact that therapeutic decisions must be made for sick patients regardless of the quality of existing evidence on the subject. In the absence of a clear-cut consensus favoring one mode of treatment over the others, various treatments are often given. As a result, in the course of ordinary patient care large numbers of patients receive various treatments and go on to manifest their effects. If experience with these patients can be captured and properly analyzed, it can be used to guide therapeutic decisions.

Unfortunately, it is often difficult to be sure that observational studies involve unbiased comparisons. Decisions about treatment are determined by a great many factors—severity of illness, concurrent diseases, local preferences, patient cooperation, etc. Patients receiving the various treatments are likely to differ not only in their treatment, but in other ways as well. Efforts to determine the results of treatment alone, free from other factors, are thereby compromised.

Example—There has been a long-standing controversy about whether anticoagulants lower the death rate from acute myocardial infarction (AMI). In a study of this question (discussed earlier), the records of 2330 patients treated for AMI in 22 hospitals were reviewed. Physicians had determined which patients received anticoagulants and which did not, using their clinical judgment.

Patients given anticoagulants had a lower 21-day mortality rate than those not receiving such therapy (8.3% versus 27.3%, $p < 0.001$). The authors noted that the difference in outcome rates did not seem related to a variety of prognostic factors, including sex, disease severity, site of infarction, diagnostic criteria, or type of hospital.

However, patients not given anticoagulants were older: 65% were at least 60 years old, whereas only 43% of patients given anticoagulants were this old. Also, patients not given anticoagulants had a much higher mortality rate within the first 48 hours of admission (12.2% versus 1.9%), before anticoagulants could be expected to exert a protective effect, suggesting that they were in general sicker. Although these two characteristics, in themselves, do not account for all the difference in mortality, they do establish that there were systematic differences in prognosis in the groups other than whether anticoagulants had been given.

Therefore, it was not possible to reach any firm conclusion in this study about the value of anticoagulants for AMI (7).

Randomization

In order to study the unique effects of a clinical intervention, the best way to allocate patients is by means of *randomization*. Patients are allocated to receive either the experimental or control treatment by one of a variety of disciplined procedures—analogous to flipping a coin—whereby each patient has an equal chance of appearing in any one of the treatment groups.

Random allocation of patients is preferable because randomization assigns patients to one group or the other(s) without bias. That is, patients in one group are, on the average, as likely to possess a given characteristic as patients in another. This is so for all factors related to prognosis, whether or not they are known before the study takes place.

In the long run, with a large number of patients in the trial, randomization usually works as described above. However, random allocation is no guarantee that the groups will be similar. Although the process of random allocation is unbiased, the results may not be. Dissimilarities between groups can arise, albeit infrequently, by chance alone. The risk of dissimilar groups is particularly great when the number of patients randomized is small. (Consider the probability, roughly one in 100, that flipping a coin 10 times will produce heads just half of the time, as opposed to getting very close to 50% heads in the long run, after 1000 tosses.)

To assess whether this kind of "bad luck" has occurred, authors of randomized controlled trials often present a table comparing the frequency of a variety of characteristics in the treated and control groups, especially those known to be related to outcome. It is reassuring to see that important characteristics have, in fact, fallen out nearly equally in the groups being compared. If they have not, it is possible to see what the differences are and attempt to control them in the analysis (Chapter 6).

Some investigators believe it is best to make sure, before randomization, that at least some of the characteristics known to be strongly associated with outcome will appear equally in treated and control groups in order to reduce the risk of bad luck. They suggest that patients first be gathered into groups (strata) of similar prognosis and then randomized separately within each stratum—a process called *stratified randomization* (Fig. 7.8). The groups are then bound to be comparable, at least for the factors that have been dealt with in this way. Others argue that whatever differences arise by bad luck are unlikely to be large and can be dealt with mathematically after the data are collected.

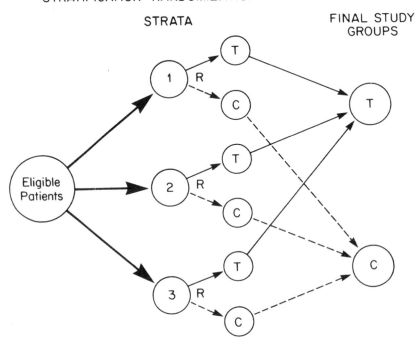

Figure 7.8. Stratified randomization: Patients are first divided into strata (1–3) according to one or more prognostic factors and then randomized separately within each stratum into treated (*T*) and control (*C*) groups.

DIFFERENCES ARISING AFTER RANDOMIZATION

Not all patients in a clinical trial receive the treatment that they were randomized to receive. Some patients drop out, do not take their medications, leave the study because of side effects or other illnesses, or somehow obtain the other treatment. Although the only difference in treatment between the two groups in the trial is supposed to be the experimental treatment, study patients often receive other treatments as well. What are the consequences of these differences, arising after randomization, and how are they dealt with?

Management and Explanatory Trials

The results of a randomized, controlled trial can be analyzed and presented in two ways: according to the treatment patients were randomized to, or the one they actually received. The correct presentation of results depends on the question being asked.

If the question is, "Which treatment policy is best, at the time the decision must be made?," then analysis according to the assigned (randomized) group is appropriate—whether or not some patients did not receive the treatment they were supposed to receive. Trials presented in this way are called *management trials* (9). The advantages of this approach are that the question corresponds to the one actually faced by clinicians and the groups compared are really randomized. The disadvantage is that, if many patients do not receive the treatment to which they were randomized, differences between experimental and control groups will tend to be obscured, increasing the chances of a negative study. Then if the study shows no difference, it is uncertain whether the treatment is truly ineffective or was just not received.

Another question is "Is the experimental treatment, if actually received, better?" For this question, the proper analysis is according to the treatment each patient actually received, regardless of the treatment to which they were randomized. Trials analyzed in this way are called *explanatory trials* because they emphasize the mechanism by which effects are exerted. The problem with this approach is that it no longer represents a randomized trial; it is simply a cohort study. Therefore, one must be concerned about dissimilarities between groups, other than the experimental treatment, and must use one or more methods (restriction, matching, stratification or adjustment) to achieve comparability, just as one would for any nonexperimental study.

Co-Interventions

After randomization, patients may receive a variety of interventions other than the ones being studied. If these occur unequally in the two groups and affect outcomes, they can introduce a bias.

Example—The Multiple Risk Factor Intervention Trial was a study of the effectiveness of a program to prevent cardiovascular disease by efforts to reduce risk factors. People without apparent cardiovascular disease, but at increased risk of developing it, were randomly allocated to enter a special program or to remain under usual medical care. The rates of cardiovascular events during the next 7 years were compared. Risk factors were reduced in the experimental group as expected. Yet, they were also reduced in the comparison group. Differences in cardiovascular disease rates between the two groups were small and not statistically significant.

Apparently, improvements in health behavior in the general population (and hence in the comparison group) and more aggressive usual medical care, perhaps stimulated by local screening and other study activities, occurring during the time of the study diminished the contrast between experimental and comparison patients so that little difference in cardiovascular disease rates was found (10).

Responders Versus Nonresponders

The results of clinical trials, particularly those about cancer, are sometimes reported according to whether patients are "responders" or "nonresponders." The outcomes of patients who initially improve after treatment ("responders") are compared to outcomes in those who do not ("nonresponders"). The implication is that one can learn something about the efficacy of treatment in this way.

This approach is scientifically unsound and often misleading because response and nonresponse might be associated with many characteristics related to the ultimate outcome: stage of disease, rate of progression, compliance, dose and side effects of drugs, the presence of other diseases, etc. If no patient actually improved because of the treatment, and patients were destined to follow various clinical courses, then some (the ones who happened to be doing well) would be called "responders" and others (the ones having a bad course) would be considered "nonresponders." Responders would, of course, have a better outcome—whether or not they received the experimental treatment.

Compliance

Compliance (discussed earlier) is another characteristic that can arise after randomization. Therefore, comparing responses among compliant and noncompliant patients in a randomized trial can be misleading.

Example—During a large study of the effects of several lipid-lowering drugs on coronary heart disease, 1103 men were given clofibrate and 2789 men were given placebo. The 5-year mortality rate was 20.0% for the clofibrate group and 20.9% for the placebo group, indicating that the drug was not effective.

It was recognized that not all patients took their medications. Was clofibrate effective among patients who actually took the drug? The answer appeared to be yes. Among patients given clofibrate, 5-year mortality for patients taking most of their prescribed drug was 15.0%, compared to 24.6% for the less cooperative patients ($p < 10^{-5}$). However, taking the prescribed drug was also related to lower mortality rates among patients prescribed placebo. For them, 5-year mortality was 15.1% for patients taking most of their placebo medication and 28.3 for patients who did not ($p < 10^{-15}$). It was apparent that there was an association between drug taking and prognosis that was not related to clofibrate.

The authors cautioned against evaluating treatment effects in subgroups determined by patient responses to the treatment protocol after randomization (11).

BLINDING

The cast of characters in a clinical trial includes three basic actors: those who give treatment (clinicians), those who receive it (patients), and those who assess its effects (investigators). Often the clinicians and investigators are the same people. Participants in a trial may change their behavior in a systematic way (i.e., be biased) if they are aware of which patients receive which treatment.

Blinding refers to any attempt to make the various participants in a study unaware of which treatment patients have been offered, so that the knowledge cannot cause them to act differently and thereby damage the internal validity of the study. "Masking" is a more appropriate metaphor, but blinding is the time-honored term.

Blinding can take place at four levels in a clinical trial. First, those responsible for allocating patients to treatment groups should not know which treatment will be assigned next so that the knowledge cannot affect their willingness to enter patients in the trial. Second, patients should be unaware of which treatment they are taking; they are thereby less likely to change their compliance or their reporting of symptoms because of this information. Third, physicians who take care of patients in the study should not know which treatment each patient has been given; then they will not, perhaps unconsciously, manage them differently. Finally, if the researchers who assess outcomes cannot distinguish treatment groups, that knowledge cannot affect their measurements. The terms "single-blind" (patients) and "double-blind" (patients and researchers) are sometimes used, but their meaning is ambiguous.

Blinding is most needed when the occurrence and reporting of the outcomes under consideration—for example, pain, nausea, or disability—can be influenced easily by knowledge of treatment. "Hard" outcomes, such as death, recurrence of cancer, or culture-positive infection, are generally less susceptible to biases resulting from knowledge of treatment.

When blinding is possible, it is usually accomplished by means of a placebo. However, for many important clinical questions—the effects of surgery, radiotherapy, diet, or the organization of medical care—blinding of patients and managing physicians is not possible.

Even when blinding appears to be possible, it is more often claimed than done. Physiologic effects, such as lowered pulse rate with beta-blocking drugs, or bone marrow depression with cancer chemotherapy, are regular features of some medications. Symptoms may also be a clue. For example, in the Lipids Research Clinics trial of the primary prevention of cardiovascular disease, a nearly perfect placebo was used. Some people received cholestyramine and others a powder of the same appearance, odor, and taste. But side effects were substantially more common in the cholestyramine group—so much so that patients might have guessed their treatment. For example, an analysis of side effects at the end of the first year of the trial showed much higher rates for the experimental (cholestyramine) group than the control group for constipation (39 versus 10%), heartburn (27 versus 10%), belching and bloating (27 versus 16%), and nausea (16 versus 8%) (12).

There is also objective evidence that patients and physicians in some blinded trials can guess who received what treatment.

Example—A double-blind, randomized trial was conducted to see if propranolol could prevent another myocardial infarction in patients who had already had one (13). At the conclusion of the trial, but before unblinding, patients and clinic personnel were asked to guess the treatment group assignment of each patient. The percentages of participants guessing correctly are shown in Table 7.2.

Clinical personnel seemed to be aided, in their guessing, by observation of heart rate; it was unclear how patients knew.

Assessment of Outcomes

In general, the more clear-cut the end points used, the less opportunity there is for bias. When the outcome of a trial is measured in unequivocal terms, such as being alive or dead, it is unlikely that patients will be misclassified, no matter how biased the assessment of outcome might be. However, for outcomes that are decided by the opinion of one of the participants, there is opportunity for bias. For example, although the fact of death is usually clear, the cause of death is often not. Most persons die for a combination of reasons or for obscure reasons, allowing some room for judgment in assigning cause of death. This judgment can be influenced by knowledge of what went before, including the treatments that were given. Opportunities for bias are even greater when assessing such symptoms as pain, nausea, or depression.

Table 7.2

Percentage of Patients and Medical Personnel Involved in a Randomized Double-Blind Controlled Trial of Propranolol Who Guessed the Treatment Group Correctly[a]

PARTICIPANT	ACTUAL TREATMENT GROUP	
	PROPRANOLOL	PLACEBO
Patient	79.9	57.2
Physician	69.9	68.8
Clinic coordinator	67.1	70.6

[a] From Byington RP, et al: Assessment of double-blindedness at the conclusion of the beta-blocker heart attack trial. *JAMA* 253:1733–1736, 1985.

CLINICAL TRIALS AND INDIVIDUAL PATIENTS

The best predictor of clinical phenomena in individual patients is past experience with groups of similar patients. To obtain this information requires pooling the experience of many patients who are admittedly dissimilar and describing what happens to them on the average. How can we obtain more precise estimates for individual patients? Three ways are to narrow the range of possible characteristics for patients in the trial (restriction), examine subgroups, or study individual patients.

Subgroups

The principal result of a clinical trial is a description of the most important outcome in each of the major treatment groups. But it is tempting to examine the results in more detail than the overall conclusions afford. We begin to look at subgroups of patients with special characteristics or for particular outcomes. In doing so, however, there are some risks that are not a feature of examining the principal conclusions alone. Trials that are large enough to answer the principal questions may be far too small to answer more detailed ones.

Example—In the VA Trial of the treatment of hypertension (diastolic blood pressure 115–129 mm Hg), there was a statistically significant reduction in morbid events in the treated groups. In all, 27 severe complicating events developed among patients given placebo and only 2 among patients given antihypertensive drugs (p < .001).

The general conclusions were accepted, but more specific questions were raised. Did treatment prevent myocardial infarctions? What about renal failure or retinopathy? These questions could not be answered with confidence because there were simply not enough patients in the study. A total of 143 treated and control patients was sufficient to answer the overall question of benefit. But when the rates of specific events were examined, comparisons involved very small numbers (Table 7.3). For example, only two untreated patients had worsening renal function, and none in the treated group; three untreated patients had dissecting aneurysms, and none of the treated; and so on.

Clearly, each of these individual findings could have easily arisen by chance, although the overall distribution of complication—27 versus 2—was very unlikely to be by chance alone (14).

Because examining subgroups in a clinical trial—either certain kinds of patients or specific kinds of outcomes—involves a great reduction in the data available, it is frequently impossible to come to firm conclusions. Nevertheless, the temptation to look is there, and some tentative information can be gleaned. Also, when subgroups are defined by characteristics arising after randomization, they should be treated like the groups of any other nonrandomized study. It is necessary to look for systematic differences in the groups being compared and correct for them if they are found.

Table 7.3

The Paucity of Data in Subgroups: The Occurrence of Severe, Complicating Events in Men With Diastolic Blood Pressure Averaging 115–129 mm Hg, Treated with Antihypertensive Drugs or Placebo[a]

EVENT	NUMBER	
	PLACEBO (N = 70)	TREATED (N = 73)
Retinopathy	9	
Heart disease	4	
Cerebrovascular disease	4	1
Increasing hypertension	3	
Aortic dissection or aneurysm	3	
Azotemia	3	
Sudden death	1	
Depression		1
Total	27	2

[a] Data from Veterans Administration Cooperative Study Group on Antihypertensive Agents: Effects of treatment on morbidity in hypertension. Results in patients with diastolic blood pressures averaging 115 through 129 mm Hg. *JAMA* 202:1028–1034, 1967.

Trials on Individual Patients

Because a treatment that is effective on the average may not work on an individual patient, the results of valid clinical research are a good reason to begin treating a patient, but experience with that patient is a better reason to continue therapy. Therefore, when conducting a treatment program it is useful to ask the following series of questions:

Is the treatment known to be efficacious for any patients?

Is the treatment known to be effective, on the average, in patients like mine?

Are the benefits worth the discomforts and risks?

Is the treatment working in my patients?

By asking these questions, one can guard against ill-founded choice of treatment or stubborn persistence in the face of poor results.

Rigorous clinical trials, with proper attention to bias and chance, can be done with individual patients, one at a time (15). The method, called *Trials of N = 1*, is an improvement in a more informal process—trial and error—that has been long used in clinical practice. A patient is given one or another treatment (e.g., active treatment or placebo) in random order, each for a brief period of time, such as a week or two. Patients and physicians are blind to which treatment is given. Outcomes—for example, a simple preference for treatment or a symptom score—are assessed after each period and subjected to statistical analysis.

This method is useful when activity of disease is unpredictable, response to treatment is prompt, and there is no carryover effect from period to period. Examples of diseases in which the method can be used include migraine, bronchospasm, fibrositis, and functional bowel disease.

Trials of $N = 1$ can be useful for guiding clinical decision making, although for a relatively small proportion of patients. They can also be used to screen interesting clinical hypotheses in order to select some that are promising enough to be evaluated using a full randomized controlled trial involving many patients.

ETHICS

Patients and physicians who become involved in clinical trials often find they are not entirely comfortable with the experience. The various trappings of sound clinical trials—control groups, random allocation of treatment, and blindness—seem like very severe constraints compared to the options available in most doctor-patient encounters, where the sole objective is patient care.

Some critics of clinical trials are concerned that patients may not be offered the best possible treatment, according to current knowledge. In fact, trials are not considered ethical if there is already good evidence that one of the treatments is superior. But if it is really not known which is better, how can it be wrong to give one treatment, rather than the other? It might even be argued that it is wrong to give a treatment that is not known to be efficacious.

A large number of safeguards have been developed so that patients do not participate in experiments against their will. Physicians have considerable power over sick people, particularly when patients are in an unusually dependent position—for example, when they are desperately ill, prisoners, or relatively unsophisticated. Also, some physicians have abused their power in the name of gaining new knowledge. How, then, can we ask patients to participate in clinical trials in a way that they can refuse and, if they accept, in a way that protects their rights?

At the present time, proposals for research involving humans must be approved by a "Committee on the Protection of Human Subjects" at the sponsoring institution. Members represent various disciplines in the institution and community and are not directly involved in the proposed research. Particular attention is given to ensuring that patients are not exposed to undue risk (relative to the usual care for their condition) and that they have given informed consent for their participation. Table 7.4 shows the elements of informed consent used at our institution. The document meets federal regulations for human research, and similar requirements are used in institutions throughout the United States.

Unfortunately, there is reason to question whether signing a consent form really means a patient has understood its stipulations. Legal documents notwithstanding, informed consent still rests largely on the ability of investigators to communicate honestly and fully with their subjects.

Table 7.4
Elements of Consent Forms for Human Subjects in Research[a]

1. Name and telephone number of Principal Investigator
2. Written in simple, easily understood language (in first person)
3. A statement that the study involves research
4. An explanation of the *purpose* of the research, *identifying procedures that are experimental*
5. An explanation of the procedures to be followed
6. The approximate number of subjects involved in the study
7. Description of benefits to be reasonably expected
8. Description of *all* discomforts and risks to be reasonably expected
9. A statement that some risks may be unforeseeable, e.g., pharmacokinetic and other studies of new drugs, devices, etc.
10. Disclosure of *any* alternative procedures that might be advantageous to the subject
11. The expected duration of the subject's participation, frequency of trips to study site, etc.
12. A statement of any costs to the subjects: clinic fees, professional fees, diagnostic and laboratory studies, drugs, devices, transportation
13. A statement describing confidentiality
14. Records may be reviewed:
    a) By FDA, if sponsored by them
    b) By manufacturers of drug or device, if sponsored by them
15. A statement that the subject is free to withdraw from the research activity at any time without penalty and without jeopardizing his or her continuing medical care at this institution
16. The following statement must be included in all Consent Forms (Federal & UNC regulations):
    I understand that in the event of physical injury directly resulting from the research procedures, financial compensation cannot be provided. However, every effort will be made to make available to me the facilities and professional skills of (institution).
17. A statement that the project has been approved by the Committee on the Protection of the Rights of Human Subjects *and* instruction that, if the subject believes that there is any infringement upon these rights, he or she may contact the Chairman of the Committee (name, telephone number)
18. Signature of the subject indicating consent (signature of parents or legal guardians for subjects who cannot legally represent themselves)
19. Signature of witness and *date*
20. When appropriate, a simply worded *assent form* for children who can read and write should be prepared for their signature. This is *in addition* to the *consent form* signed by the parent or guardian.

[a] Adapted from the form in use at the University of North Carolina.

Acceptance Before Evidence

Not infrequently, treatments become firmly ensconced in our therapeutic armamentarium before they have been subjected to sound evaluation by means of controlled clinical trials. This problem is less likely to occur for new drugs, because the Food and Drug Administration requires evidence of safety and efficacy before licensing pharmaceuticals. However, new technology and surgical procedures are not subject to much regulation and often come into general use before controlled clinical trials have been undertaken. In fact, new procedures can become so much a part of usual practice that it is virtually impossible to conduct a trial of them. Examples of treatments that have become conventional in the absence of controlled trials include coronary care units, radical mastectomy, and caesarian section for fetal distress.

Because of this problem, some physicians have advocated "randomization from the first patient" after a new treatment is introduced. Others argue that it is better to conduct rigorous clinical trials somewhat later, after the best way to deliver the treatment has been worked out, so that a good example of the intervention is tested. In any case, it is generally agreed that if a controlled trial is postponed too long, the opportunity to do it at all may be lost.

Clinical trials are undoubtedly awkward to conduct. But as a society, we have little choice. If some patients do not participate in trials, then all patients will be treated without the best possible evidence that more good than harm is being accomplished.

THE REAL WORLD

Randomized, controlled, blinded trials are the standard of excellence for comparisons of effects over time. A properly designed trial, even if it is impossible to carry out, can be used as a point of reference to design or judge the validity of observational studies (cohort or case-control studies) of the same question. To the extent that observational studies must stray from the experimental design, we should be concerned about their validity and estimate the effects of the bias.

This does not mean that only clinical trials should be done for all questions of cause and effect. They cannot. It is not ethical to assign potentially harmful exposures to people deliberately, however important the question. So clinical trials cannot be used to study the causes of disease. Also, trials of some potentially helpful interventions may not be possible for such practical reasons as cost, delay in obtaining the results, or the number of patients available. Because of these many practical difficulties with randomized controlled clinical trials, the majority of therapeutic questions are answered by other means, particularly uncontrolled and nonrandomized trials.

Partly for a lack of substantial evidence, there remains a great deal of controversy about the value of many everyday clinical treatments. There has been vigorous, sometimes acrimonious debate over the effects of "tight" blood sugar control on the chronic complications of diabetes, the value of streptokinase after acute myocardial infarction, and the best surgical procedure for breast cancer—to name just a few.

Although randomized controlled trials are certainly expensive and difficult, their alternative—patient care without sound guidelines—may be more so. Each year, billions of dollars are spent on diagnostic and therapeutic efforts that are of uncertain value. Under the circumstances, properly designed and timely clinical trials could save money.

SUMMARY

Promising ideas about what might be good treatment should be put to a rigorous test before being accepted. The best test is a randomized controlled trial, a special case of a cohort study in which the intervention is allocated without bias. Patients in clinical trials are usually highly selected, reducing generalizability. They are randomly allocated to receive either an experimental intervention or some comparison management: usual treatment, a placebo, or simple observation. On the average, the compared groups have a similar prognosis just after randomization (and before the interventions), but differences not attributable to treatment can arise later, including dropouts and crossovers, co-interventions, and non-compliance. Blinding all participants in the trial can help to minimize bias.

For many questions it is not possible to have a concurrent, randomized control group and blinding. Compromises with the ideal include making comparisons to experience with past patients, to past experience with the same patients, or to a concurrent group of patients who are not randomly allocated. When this is done, the internal validity of the study is weakened.

Figure 7.9 indicates principal locations of potential bias in randomized controlled trials:

1. What kinds of patients are considered for the trial?
2. Are the patients who are actually studied an unbiased sample of all patients with the condition?
3. Are patients allocated to study groups without bias?
4. To what management is the experimental intervention compared?

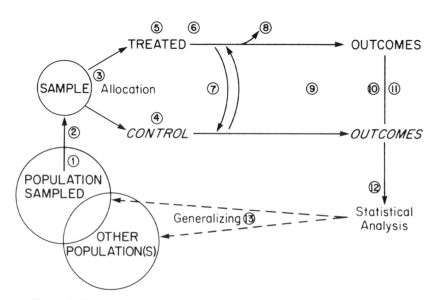

Figure 7.9. Locations of potential bias in a randomized controlled trial.

5. What is the experimental intervention?
6. Were patients compliant with the intervention?
7. Did patients cross over between treatment groups after randomization?
8. Did patients drop out of the study after randomization?
9. Were there interventions other than the ones being studied?
10. Are the outcomes important in human terms?
11. Were the outcomes sought with equal vigor and defined by similar criteria in the two groups?
12. Could the observed results have happened by chance alone?
13. To whom do the results apply?

REFERENCES

1. Thomas L:Biostatistics in medicine. *Science* 198:675, 1977.
2. The EC/IC Bypass Study Group: Failure of extracranial-intracranial arterial bypass to reduce the risk of ischemic stroke. *N Engl J Med* 313:1191–1200, 1985.
3. Opie on the heart. *Lancet* 1:692, 1980.
4. CASS Principal Investigators and their Associates: Coronary Artery Surgery Study (CASS): a randomized trial of coronary artery bypass surgery. Survival data. *Circulation* 68:939–950, 1983.
5. Hill JD, Hampton JR, Mitchell JRA: A randomized trial of home versus hospital management for patients with suspected acute myocardial infarction. *Lancet* 1:837–841, 1978.
6. Sacks H, Chalmers TC, Smith H Jr: Randomized versus historical controls for clinical trials. *Am J Med* 72:233–240, 1982.
7. Modan B, Shani M, Schor S, Modan M: Reduction of hospital mortality from acute myocardial infarction by anticoagulant therapy. *N Engl J Med* 292:1359–1362, 1975.
8. Fischer RW: Comparison of antipruritic drugs administered orally. *JAMA* 203:418–419, 1968.
9. Sackett DL, Gent M: Controversy in counting and attributing events in clinical trials. *N Engl J Med* 301:1410–1412, 1979.
10. Multiple Risk Factor Intervention Trial Research Group: Multiple risk factor intervention trial. *JAMA* 248:1465–1477, 1982.
11. The Coronary Drug Project Research Group: Influence of adherence to treatment and response of cholesterol on mortality in the coronary drug project. *N Engl J Med* 303:1038–1041, 1980.
12. Lipid Research Clinics Program: The Lipid Research Clinics coronary primary prevention trial results. 1. Reduction in incidence of coronary heart disease. *JAMA* 251:351–364, 1984.
13. Byington RP, Curb JD, Mattson ME, et al: Assessment of double-blindness at the conclusion of the beta-blocker heart attack trial. *JAMA* 253:1733–1736, 1985.
14. Veterans Administration Cooperative Study Group on Antihypertensive Agents: Effects of treatment on morbidity in hypertension. Results in patients with diastolic blood pressures averaging 115 through 129 mm Hg. *JAMA* 202:1028–1034, 1967.
15. Guyatt G, Sackett D, Taylor DW, Chong J, Roberts R, Pugsley S: Determining optimal therapy—randomized trials in individual patients. *N Engl J Med* 314:889–892, 1986.

SUGGESTED READINGS

Chalmers TC: A potpourri of RCT topics. *Controlled Clin Trials* 3:285–298, 1982.
Chalmers TC, Smith H Jr, Blackburn B, Silverman B, Schroeder B, Reitman D, Ambroz A: A method for assessing the quality of a randomized control trial. *Controlled Clin Trials* 2:31–49, 1981.
Chalmers TC, Celano P, Sacks HS, Smith H Jr: Bias in treatment assignment in controlled clinical trials. *N Engl J Med* 309:1358–1361, 1983.

Department of Clinical Epidemiology and Biostatistics, McMaster University, Hamilton, Ontario: How to read clinical journals V: To distinguish useful from useless or even harmful therapy. *Can Med Assoc J* 124:1156–1162, 1981.

DerSimonian R, Charette LJ, McPeek B, Mosteller F: Reporting on methods in clinical trials. *N Engl J Med* 306:1332–1337, 1982.

Friedman LM, Furberg CD, DeMets DL: *Fundamentals of Clinical Trials*, ed 2. Littleton, MA, John Wright PSG Inc, 1985.

Guyatt G, Sackett D, Taylor DW, Chong J, Roberts R, Pugsley S: Determining optimal therapy—randomized trials in individual patients. *N Engl J Med* 314:889–892, 1986.

Lavori PW, Louis TA, Bailar JC III, Polansky M: Design for experiments—parallel comparisons of treatment. *N Engl J Med* 309:1291–1298, 1983.

Mantel N: An uncontrolled clinical trial—treatment response or spontaneous improvement? *Controlled Clin Trials* 3:369–370, 1982.

Meinert CL: *Clinical Trials. Design, Conduct and Analysis.* New York, Oxford University Press, 1986.

Mosteller F, Gilbert JP, McPeek B: Reporting standards and research strategies for controlled trials. *Controlled Clin Trials* 1:37–58, 1980.

Oye RK, Shapiro MF: Reporting results from chemotherapy trials. Does response make a difference in patient survival? *JAMA* 252:2722–2725, 1984.

Peto R, Pike MC, Armitage P, Breslow NE, Cox DR, Howard SV, Mantel N, McPherson K, Peto J, Smith PG: Design and analysis of randomized clinical trials requiring prolonged observation of each patient. *Br J Cancer* 34:585–612, 1976; 35:1–39, 1977.

Pocock SJ: *Clinical Trials. A Practical Approach.* New York, John Wiley and Sons, 1983.

Schwartz D, Flamant R, Lellouch J: *Clinical Trials.* New York, Academic Press, 1980.

Spilker B: *Guide to Clinical Studies and Developing Protocols.* New York, Raven Press, 1984.

Weiss GB, Bunce H III, Hokanson JA: Comparing survival of responders and nonresponders after treatment: A potential source of confusion in interpreting cancer clinical trials. *Controlled Clin Trials* 4:43–52, 1983.

chapter 8

PREVENTION

Live sensibly—among a thousand
people, only one dies a natural
death, the rest succumb to
irrational modes of living.

Maimonides
1135–1204

Most doctors are attracted to medicine because they look forward to curing disease. But all things considered, most patients would prefer never to contract a disease in the first place—or, if they must contract an illness, they prefer that it be caught early and stamped out before it causes them any harm. To accomplish this, procedures are sometimes performed on patients without specific complaints, to identify risk factors or find disease early in its course, so that by intervening, patients can remain well. Such activity is referred to as the *periodic health examination*.

Periodic health examinations constitute a large portion of clinical practice; in a national survey of ambulatory care in the United States, they were the most common reason for office visits to family practitioners, pediatricians, and obstetrician-gynecologists; the fourth most common for internists; and the sixth most common for surgeons (1). Physicians should, therefore, have some understanding about the content of the periodic health examination. They should be prepared to answer such questions as "Why do I have to get a Pap smear again this year, doctor?" or "My neighbor gets a chest x-ray every year; why aren't you ordering one for me?"

Many of the principles of the scientific approach to prevention in clinical medicine, particularly the principles underlying the use of diagnostic tests, determination of disease prognosis, and determination of the effect of intervention, have already been covered in this book. This chapter will expand on those principles and strategies as they specifically relate to prevention.

LEVELS OF PREVENTION

The dictionary defines prevention as "the act of keeping from happening" (2). With this definition in mind, almost all activities in medicine could be defined as prevention. After all, clinicians' efforts are aimed at preventing the untimely occurrences of the 6 Ds: death, disease, disability, discomfort, dissatisfaction, and destitution (Chapter 1).

Depending on when the clinical efforts are made, three types of prevention are usually possible (Fig. 8.1).

Primary prevention keeps disease from occurring at all by removing risk factors. Immunizations for many communicable diseases are examples of this kind of prevention, as is helping people to stop smoking. *Secondary prevention* detects disease early when it is still asymptomatic and when early treatment can stop the disease from progressing; pap smears and other tests for occult malignancies are examples. *Tertiary prevention* refers to those clinical activities that prevent further deterioration or reduce complications after a disease has declared itself. An example is the use of beta-blocking drugs to decrease the risk of death in patients who have recovered from myocardial infarction.

Primary prevention is often accomplished outside the health care system. Chlorination and fluoridation of the water supply and laws mandating seat belt use in automobiles and helmets for motorcycle use are examples of community-wide primary prevention programs. Other primary prevention activities occur in specific occupational settings (use of earplugs or dust masks), in schools (visual acuity tests), or in specialized health care settings (use of tests to detect the hepatitis B or the AIDS virus in blood banks). There are fewer community-wide programs in secondary prevention (shopping mall fairs for glaucoma screening are an example) and few, if any, tertiary prevention programs outside the health care system.

Physicians' practices traditionally are the mirror image of the above. Most effort is spent on tertiary prevention, less on secondary prevention, and least on primary prevention. Nevertheless, as pointed out above, a substantial proportion of office practices in pediatrics, OB-Gyn, family practice, and internal medicine is devoted to primary and secondary prevention through such activities as prenatal and well-child care, immu-

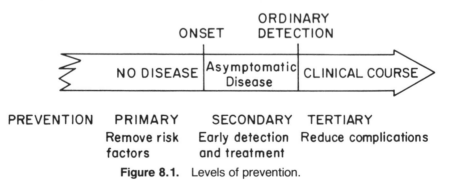

Figure 8.1. Levels of prevention.

nizations, lifestyle counseling, and screening for early disease or risk factors.

SCREENING AND CASE FINDING

Screening has been defined as

the presumptive identification of an unrecognized disease or defect by the application of tests, examinations, or other procedures which can be applied rapidly. . . . Screening tests sort out apparently well persons who have a disease from those who probably do not. A screening test is not intended to be diagnostic. Persons with positive or suspicious findings must be referred to their physicians for diagnosis and treatment (3).

When screening tests are applied to large, unselected populations, the process is called *mass screening.* Blood pressure measurements on passers-by in a shopping mall are an example of mass screening. Clinicians, on the other hand, use screening tests in a different context. Their concern about unrecognized disease is for their own patients and not so much for the population at large. *Case finding* occurs when clinicians search for disease with screening tests among their own patients who are consulting them for unrelated symptoms.

The distinction between mass screening and case finding is subtle but important. In the shopping mall, those examining the patient have no personal responsibility for following up abnormal results with appropriate diagnosis and treatment. Instead, the patient is referred to his or her doctor for further management. Many studies have shown inadequate follow-up among people with abnormalities found in mass screening. On the other hand, in case finding the clinician has the explicit responsibility for follow-up of abnormal results. If the clinician is not committed to further investigation of abnormal results and treatment if necessary, the test should not be performed at all.

WHICH DISEASES?

When considering which screening tests to perform routinely on asymptomatic patients, a decision first must be made as to which medical problems or diseases should be sought. This statement is so straightforward that it would seem unnecessary. But the fact is that many screening tests are performed without any clear understanding of what is being sought. For instance, a urinalysis is frequently ordered by physicians performing routine checkups on their patients. However, a urinalysis might be used to search for any number of medical problems, including diabetes, asymptomatic urinary tract infections, and renal calculi. It is necessary to decide which, if any, of these conditions is worth screening for before undertaking the test.

Three criteria are important when deciding which medical condition should be sought during screening (Table 8.1): (a) the effectiveness of the

Table 8.1

Criteria for Deciding whether a Medical Condition should be Sought During Periodic Health Examinations

1. If the condition is found, how effective is the ensuing treatment in terms of:
    Efficacy
    Patient compliance
    Early treatment more effective than later treatment
2. How great is the burden of suffering caused by the condition in terms of:
    Death   Discomfort
    Disease   Dissatisfaction
    Disability   Destitution
3. How good is the screening procedure in terms of:
    Sensitivity   Cost   Labeling effects
    Specificity   Safety
    Simplicity   Acceptability

ensuing treatment if the condition is found, (b) the burden of suffering caused by the condition, and (c) the accuracy of the screening test.

Effectiveness of Early Treatment

The most important question to ask before screening for a medical condition is whether or not earlier treatment is effective. If early treatment is not effective, it is not worth searching for the medical problem regardless of how easily it can be found, because early detection alone merely extends the length of time the disease is known to exist, without helping the patient.

This principle is illustrated by a study of the use of chest x-rays to screen for lung cancer. People who were screened every 6 months with x-ray examinations and treated promptly if cancer was found did no better than those not offered x-rays; at 5 years, less than 10% of patients with lung cancer were alive in either group (4). Early detection and treatment, therefore, did not help patients with lung cancer.

Effectiveness of treatment is covered in detail in Chapter 7. In the context of screening, for a treatment to be effective, these conditions must be met: (a) The treatment itself must work (efficacy), (b) patients must accept the treatment (patient compliance), and (c) the results of treatment must be better early in the course of disease, when it is asymptomatic, than later after the condition becomes symptomatic and is discovered because the person seeks medical care.

As discussed in Chapter 7, the best way to establish the efficacy of treatment is with a randomized controlled trial. This is true for all therapy, but is especially true for early treatment after screening. Often preventive therapy takes years to demonstrate an effect and requires large numbers of people to be studied. For example, early treatment after breast cancer screening can decrease breast cancer deaths by approximately one-third in older women. But to show this effect, a study lasting 16 years and involving more than 50,000 women was required (5). A "clinical impression" of the effect of screening simply could not suffice in this situation.

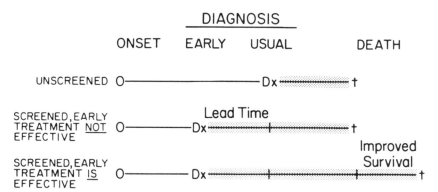

Figure 8.2. How lead time affects survival time after screening; *shaded areas* indicate length of survival.

Biases

Careful studies are also necessary because of specific biases that can occur in screening programs. Three such biases are described below.

Lead time is the period of time between the detection of a medical condition by screening and when it ordinarily would have been diagnosed because an individual experienced symptoms and sought medical care (Fig. 8.2). The amount of lead time for a given disease is dependent on both the biologic rate of progression of the disease and on the ability of the screening test to detect early disease. When lead time is very short, as is presently the case with lung cancer, the treatment of medical conditions picked up on screening is likely to be no more effective than treatment after symptoms appear. On the other hand, when lead time is long, as is true for cervical cancer (on average, it takes approximately 30 years to progress from carcinoma in situ to clinically invasive disease), the treatment of the medical condition found on screening can be very effective.

How can lead time cause biased results in a study of the efficacy of early treatment? As Figure 8.2 shows, because lead time allows a disease to be found earlier than would be the usual case, people who are diagnosed by screening for a deadly disease will, on average, live longer from the time of diagnosis than people who are diagnosed after they get symptoms, even if there is no effective treatment. It could appear that screening helps people live longer, when in a reality they have been given not more "survival time" but more "disease time."

An appropriate method of analysis to avoid lead time bias is to study both a screened group of people and a comparable control group of people and compare age-specific mortality rates, rather than survival rates from the time of diagnosis. We can be confident that early diagnoses and treatment of breast cancer is effective, because breast cancer mortality rates of screened women over age 50 are lower than those of a comparable group of unscreened women.

Another bias that can affect studies of screening, called *length/time bias*

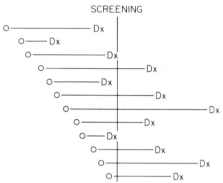

Figure 8.3. Length/time bias. Cases that progress rapidly from onset (O) to symptoms and diagnosis (Dx) are less likely to be detected during a screening examination.

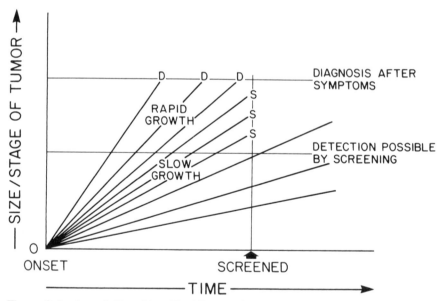

Figure 8.4. Length/time bias: Rapidly growing tumors come to medical attention before screening, whereas more slowly growing tumors are detected by screening. *D* = diagnosis after symptoms, *S* = diagnosis after screening.

(Figs. 8.3 and 8.4), occurs because the proportion of slow-growing lesions diagnosed during screening programs is greater than the proportion of those diagnosed during usual medical care. The effect of including a greater number of slow-growing cancers makes it seem that the screening and early treatment program are more effective.

Length/time bias occurs in the following way. Screening works best when a medical condition develops slowly. Most types of cancers, however, demonstrate a wide range of growth patterns. Some cancers grow slowly, some very fast. Screening tests are likely to find mostly slow-growing tumors; fast-growing ones more likely will have already caused symptoms that led to diagnosis in the interval between screening examinations. Screening, therefore, tends to find tumors with inherently the better prognosis, whereas regular care finds those with worse prognoses, even if the prognoses of each are unchanged by subsequent treatment. As a result, the mortality rates of cancers found on screening may appear better than those not found on screening, but it is not because of the screening itself.

The third major type of bias than can occur in studies of the effectiveness of early treatment is due to patient *compliance*, the extent to which patients follow medical advice. If a study compares disease outcomes among volunteers for a screening program with outcomes in a group of people who did not volunteer, better results for the volunteers might not be due to treatment, but to other differences between the two groups of patients.

Example—Bias due to patient compliance was demonstrated in a study of the effect of a health maintenance program (6). One group of patients was invited yearly for a periodic health examination, and a comparable group was not invited. Over the years, however, some of the control group asked for periodic health examinations. As seen in Figure 8.5, those patients in the control group who actively sought out the examinations had better mortality rates than the patients who were invited for screening. The latter group contained not only highly compliant patients but also ones who had to be "dragged in" as well.

Biases due to length/time and patient compliance can be avoided by relying on randomized controlled trials that count all the outcomes in the groups, regardless of the method of diagnosis or degree of participation. Groups of patients that are randomly allocated will have comparable numbers of slow and fast-growing tumors and will have, on the average, comparable levels of compliance. These groups then can be followed over time with mortality rates, rather than survival rates (to avoid lead time bias).

Burden of Suffering

The second question to ask when deciding whether to screen for a given medical condition is: Is screening justified by the severity of the medical condition in terms of mortality, morbidity, and suffering caused by the condition?

Only conditions posing threats to life or health (the 6 D's) should be sought. The severity of the medical condition is determined primarily by the risk it poses or its prognosis (discussed in Chapters 5 and 6). For example, the health consequences of asymptomatic bacteriuria are still unclear. We do not know if it causes renal failure and/or hypertension. Even so, bacteriuria is frequently sought in periodic health examinations.

A particularly difficult dilemma faced by clinicians and patients is the

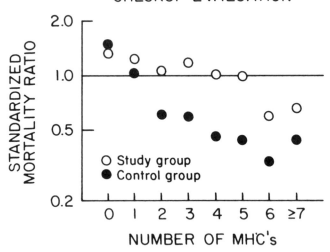

Figure 8.5. Effect of patient compliance on a screening program: the control group of patients had a lower standardized mortality ratio (observed to expected deaths, standardized for age) than the study group offered screening, but the control group included only patients who requested screening, whereas the study group included all patients offered screening. *MHC's* = Multiphasic Health Checkups. (Redrawn from Friedman GD, Collen MF, Fireman BH: Multiphasic health checkup evaluation: a 16-year follow-up. *J Chron Dis* 39:453–63, 1986.)

situation in which a person is known to be at high risk for a condition, but there is no evidence that early treatment is effective. What should the physician and patient do? For example, there is evidence that people with Barrett's esophagus (a condition in which the squamous mucosa in the distal esophagus is replaced by columnar epithelium) run a 30- to 40-fold greater risk of developing esophageal cancer than persons without Barrett's esophagus. However, the effect of screening such people with periodic endoscopic examinations followed by early treatment if cancer occurs is unknown.

There is no easy answer to this dilemma. But if physicians remember that screening will not work unless early therapy is effective, they can weigh carefully the evidence about therapy. If the evidence is against effectiveness, they are not helping their patients by screening.

WHICH TESTS?

With appropriate answers to the previous two questions, we can turn to criteria for the test itself. A screening test can be a history question ("Do you smoke?"), a part of the physical examination (a clinical breast examination), a procedure (sigmoidoscopy), or a laboratory test (hematocrit).

The following criteria for a good screening test apply equally to all types of tests.

Sensitivity and Specificity

The very nature of searching for disease in asymptomatic people means the prevalence of a particular disease is usually very low, even among high risk groups selected because of age, sex, and other characteristics. A good screening test must therefore have a high sensitivity, in order not to miss the few cases of disease that are present, and a high specificity, to reduce the number of people with false positive results who require further workup.

Because of the low prevalence of most diseases, the positive predictive value of screening tests is likely to be low, regardless of how specific a given test is. Clinicians who want to practice preventive health care by performing periodic health examinations on their patients, therefore, must accept the fact that they will have to work up many patients who will not have disease. However, they can minimize the problem by concentrating their screening efforts on people with a higher prevalence for disease.

Example—The incidence of breast cancer increases with age, from approximately 1 in 300,000/year under age 30 to 1 in 300/year over age 70. Therefore, a lump found during screening in a young woman's breast is very likely to be nonmalignant, whereas the lump in an older woman is much more likely to be malignant. In a large demonstration project on breast cancer screening, biopsy results of breast masses varied markedly according to the age of women; in women under age 40, more than 16 benign lesions were found for every malignancy, but in women over age 70 fewer than 3 benign lesions were found for every malignancy (Fig. 8.6) (7).

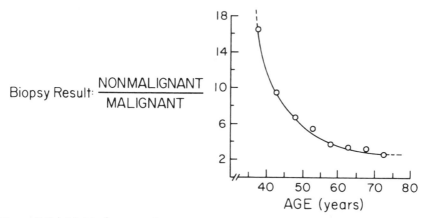

Biopsy Result: $\dfrac{NONMALIGNANT}{MALIGNANT}$

Figure 8.6.   Yield of a screening test according to patients' age: ratio of nonmalignant to malignant biopsy results among women screened for breast cancer. (Data from Baker LH: Breast Cancer Detection Demonstration Project: five-year summary report. *CA* 32:195–231, 1982.)

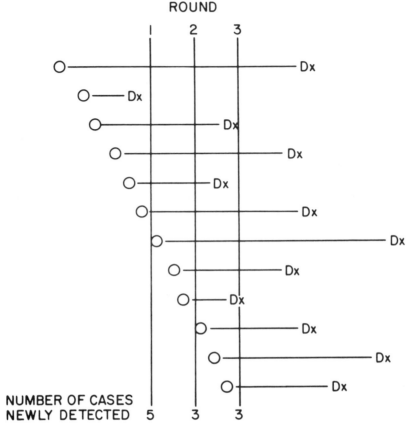

Figure 8.7. The decreasing yield of a screening test after the first round of screening. The first round (prevalence screening) detects prevalent cases. The second and third rounds (incidence screenings) detect incident cases. It is assumed that the test detects all cases and that all people in the population are screened. If not, cases not detected in the first round are available for detection in subsequent rounds—and the yield can be higher.

The problem of a low positive predictive value increases the longer that screening is carried on in a group of people. Figure 8.7 demonstrates why this is true. The first time that screening is carried out—the *prevalence screen*—cases of the medical condition will have been present for varying lengths of time. During the second round of screening, most cases found will have had their onset between the first and second screening. (A few will have been missed by the first screen.) Therefore, second and subsequent screenings are called *incidence screens*. Figure 8.7 illustrates how, when a group of people are periodically rescreened, the number of cases of disease present in the group drops after the prevalence screen. This means that the positive predictive value for test results will decrease after the first round of screening.

Simplicity and Low Cost

An ideal screening test should take only a few minutes to perform, require minimum preparation by the patient, depend on no special appointments, and be inexpensive.

Simple, quick examinations, such as blood pressure determinations, are ideal screening tests. Conversely, complicated diagnostic tests, such as barium enemas that require special diet, an x-ray appointment, bowel preparation, and discomfort during the procedure, may be reasonable in patients with symptoms and clinical indications, but are clearly unacceptable as screening tests. Other tests, such as visual field testing for the detection of glaucoma and audiograms for the detection of hearing loss, fall between these two extremes. Even if done carefully, such tests, although not as difficult as barium enemas, are probably too complex to be used as screening tests.

The financial "cost" of the test depends not only on the cost of (or charge for) the procedure itself but also on the cost of subsequent evaluations performed on patients with positive test results. Thus, sensitivity, specificity, and predictive value affect cost. Cost is also affected by whether the test requires a special visit to the physician. Screening tests performed while the patient is seeing his or her physician for other reasons (as is frequently the case with blood pressure measurements) are much cheaper for patients than tests requiring special visits, extra time off from work, and additional transportation.

Safety

Although it is reasonable and ethical to accept certain risks for diagnostic tests applied to sick patients seeking help for specific complaints, it is quite another matter to subject presumably well people to such risks. Thus, although sigmoidoscopy using a rigid sigmoidoscope is hardly thought of as a "dangerous" procedure when used on patients with gastrointestinal complaints, some reviewers have suggested it is too dangerous to use as a screening procedure because of the possibility of bowel perforation. In fact, it has been estimated that if rigid sigmoidoscopy were used to screen for colerectal cancer, as many as four perforations would occur for every cancer found (8).

Acceptable to Both Patients and Clinicians

The importance of this criterion is illustrated by experience with tests for early cervical cancer and early colon cancer. It turns out that women at greatest risk for cervical cancer are least likely to get routine pap smears. The same problem holds true for colorectal cancer. Studies indicate there is a strong reluctance among asymptomatic North Americans to submit to periodic examinations of their lower gastrointestinal tracts—a finding that should be no surprise to any of us!

Table 8.2 illustrates the problem of patients' acceptance of screening for colorectal cancer. People who were attending a colorectal cancer screening clinic were very cooperative; they were willing to collect stool samples, smear the samples on guaiac-impregnated paper slides, and mail the slides to their doctors for clinical testing. Less selected patients, however, were less willing to participate. Retired persons, who were at greatest risk for colorectal cancer because of their age, were least willing to be screened.

The acceptability of the test to clinicians is a criterion usually overlooked by all but the ones performing the test. After one large and well-conducted study on the usefulness of screening, sigmoidoscopy was abandoned because the physicians performing the procedure—gastroenterologists, at that—found it too cumbersome and time-consuming to be justified by the yield (9). (Patient acceptance, 38%, was not good either.)

The "Labeling" Effect

The *labeling* effect describes the psychological impact of test results or diagnoses on patients. Labeling effects have not been extensively studied, but the work that has been done suggests that test results can sometimes have important psychological effects on patients.

Theoretically, a labeling effect can work in either a positive or negative direction. A positive labeling effect may occur when a patient is told that all the screening test results were normal. Most clinicians have heard such responses as, "Great, that means I can keep working for another year." If being given a clean bill of health promotes a continued positive attitude towards one's daily activities, a positive labeling effect has occurred.

On the other hand, being told that something is abnormal may have an adverse psychological effect. In one study, steelworkers who were told for the first time that they had hypertension experienced a threefold increase in absenteeism, an increase that could not be explained by the medical condition itself. The authors suggested that newly labeled patients "adopt the 'sick role' and treat themselves as more 'fragile'" (10). This negative labeling effect is particularly worrisome if it occurs among patients with

Table 8.2

Patients' Acceptance of Screening Tests: Reported Response Rates for Returning Guaiac-impregnated Slides in Different Settings[a]

SETTING	PARTICIPANTS RETURNING AT LEAST ONE SLIDE
	%
Colorectal cancer screening program	85
Breast cancer screening program	70
American Association of Retired Persons chapter meetings	29

[a] From Fletcher SW, Dauphinee WD: *Clin Invest Med* 4:23–31, 1981.

false positive tests, and false positive tests are particularly likely when screening because of the low prevalence of disease. In such situations screening efforts might do more harm that good.

The Risk of a False Positive Result

The previous discussion applies to each of the individual screening tests that a clinician might consider performing during a periodic health examination. However, most clinicians do not perform only one or two tests on patients presenting for routine checkups. In one study, practicing internists believed that 57 different tests should be performed during periodic health examinations (11). Modern technology has fueled this propensity to "cover all the bases." Automated blood tests allow physicians to order up to several dozen tests with a few checks in the appropriate boxes.

When the measurements of screening tests are expressed on interval scales (as most are) and when normal is defined by the range covered by 95% of the results (as is usual), the more tests the clinician orders, the greater the risk of a false positive result. In fact, as Table 8.3 shows, if the physician orders enough tests a new abnormality will be discovered in virtually all healthy patients.

CURRENT RECOMMENDATIONS

The search for disease and risk factors in presumably healthy patients is far more complex than was once thought. Because of these complexities, current recommendations on the periodic health examination are quite different from those of the past. Several groups have recommended abandoning routine annual checkups in favor of a selective approach in which the tests to be done depend on a person's age and sex (thus, increasing prevalence). They have also tended to recommend fewer tests than previously (thus, decreasing the percentage of patients with false positive results). They have turned their attention to the selection process for deciding what medical conditions should be sought. Finally, there is an increasing concern for clear delineation of the standards that tests should meet before they are incorporated into periodic health examinations.

Table 8.3
Relation between Number of Tests Ordered and Percentage of Normal People with at Least one Abnormal Test Result[a]

NUMBER OF TESTS	PEOPLE WITH AT LEAST ONE ABNORMALITY
	%
1	5
5	23
20	64
100	99.4

[a] From Sackett DL: Clinical diagnosis and the clinical laboratory. *Clin Invest Med* 1:37–43, 1978.

Even for clinicians committed to health promotion and disease prevention, it is difficult to remember what task should be done during a particular visit by a patient, because the required tests and procedures vary according to the patient's age, sex and risks. Prompting systems, such as flow sheets in each patient's record or computerized reminders, have been shown to increase the performance of preventive procedures. These strategies maximize the potential benefit of preventive health care.

SUMMARY

Disease can be prevented by keeping it from occurring in the first place (primary prevention) or by early detection at a time when treatment is more effective (secondary prevention). "Screening," a secondary preventive activity, is often carried out in the context of a periodic health examination. Diseases are sought if early treatment is more effective than treatment at the usual time, if the disease causes a substantial burden of suffering, and if a good screening test is available.

Three potential biases threaten studies of the effectiveness of early treatment: failure to account for the lead time gained by early detection, the tendency to detect a disproportionate number of slowly advancing cases when screening prevalent cases, and confounding the good prognosis associated with compliance with the effects of the preventive intervention itself.

Screening tests should be sensitive enough to pick up most cases, specific enough that there are not too many false positive results, inexpensive, safe, and well accepted. Based on these criteria, a limited number of tests, according to age and sex, are recommended as part of a periodic health examination.

REFERENCES

1. *Medical Practice in the United States. Special Report, 1981,* The Robert Wood Johnson Foundation, PO Box 2316, Princeton, NJ, 08543-2316.
2. *Webster's New Collegiate Dictionary.* Merrion Company, Springfield, MA, 1981.
3. *Commission on Chronic Illness, Chronic Illness in the United States, vol. 1.* Cambridge, MA: Harvard University Press, 1957.
4. Brett, GZ: The value of lung cancer detection by six-monthly chest radiographs. *Thorax* 23:414–420, 1968.
5. Shapiro S, Venet W, Strax P, Venet L, Rosner R: Selection, follow-up and analysis in the Health Insurance Plan Study: a randomized trial with breast cancer screening. Selection, Follow-up and Analysis in Prospective Studies: A Workshop. *National Cancer Institute Monograph* 67, May 1985, pp 65–74.
6. Friedman GD, Collen MF, Fireman BH: Multiphasic health checkup evaluation: a 16-year follow-up. *J Chron Dis* 39:453–463, 1986.
7. Baker LH: Breast Cancer Detection Demonstration Project: five-year summary report. *CA* 32:195–231, 1982.
8. Frame PS, Carlson SJ: A clinical review of periodic health screening using specific screening criteria: Part 2. Selected endocrine, metabolic and gastrointestinal diseases. *J Fam Pract* 2:123–129, 1975.
9. Dales LG, Friedman GD, Collen MF: Evaluating periodic multiphasic health check-ups: a controlled trial. *J Chron Dis* 32:385–404, 1979.

10. Haynes RB, Sackett DL, Taylor DW, Gibson ES, Johnson AL: Increased absenteeism from work after detection and labeling of hypertensive patients. *N Engl J Med* 299:741–744, 1978.
11. Romm FJ, Fletcher SW, Hulka BS: The periodic health examination: comparison of recommendations and internists' performance. *South Med J* 74:265–271, 1981.

SUGGESTED READINGS

American Cancer Society: Report on the cancer-related health checkup. *CA* 30:194, 1980.

Canadian Task Force on the Periodic Health Examination: The periodic health examination: *Can Med Assoc J* 130:1276–1292, 1984.

Canadian Task Force on the Periodic Health Examination: Cervical cancer screening programs: summary of the 1982 Canadian Task Force report. *Can Med Assoc J* 127:581–589, 1982.

Eddy DM: *Screening for Cancer: Theory, Analysis and Design.* Englewood Cliffs, NJ: Prentice-Hall, 1980.

McDonald CJ, Hui SL, Smith DM, Tierney WM, Cohen SJ, Weinberger M, McCabe GP: Reminders to physicians from an introspective computer medical record. A two-year randomized trial. *Ann Intern Med* 100:130–138, 1984.

Miller AB (ed): *Screening for Cancer.* Orlando, FL, Academic Press, 1985.

chapter 9

CHANCE

When clinicians attempt to learn from clinical experience, whether during formal research or in the course of patient care, their efforts are impeded by two processes: bias and chance.

As we have discussed, bias is systematic error—the results of any process that causes observations to differ systematically from the true values. In clinical research, a great deal of the effort is aimed at avoiding bias where possible and dealing with bias when it is unavoidable. It is at least theoretically possible to design research that avoids bias altogether—for example, by a perfect double-blind, randomized, placebo-controlled trial.

Random error, on the other hand, is inherent in all observations. It can be minimized but never avoided altogether. Random variation can arise from either the process of measurement itself or the biologic phenomenon being measured. This source of error is called "random" because on the average it is as likely to result in observed values being on one side of the true value as on the other.

Most of us tend to overestimate the importance of chance, compared to bias, when interpreting data. We might say, in essence, "If p is <0.001, a little bit of bias can't do much harm!" But if data are assembled with unrecognized bias, no amount of statistical elegance can save the day. As one scholar put it, perhaps taking an extreme position, "A well designed, carefully executed study usually gives results that are obvious without a formal analysis and if there are substantial flaws in design or execution a formal analysis will not help" (1).

In this chapter, chance will be discussed in the context of a controlled clinical trial because that is a simple way of presenting the concepts. However, it should be noted that application of the concepts is not limited to comparisons of treatments in clinical trials. Statistics are used whenever one makes inferences about populations based on information obtained from samples.

RANDOM ERROR

When a clinical trial is conducted, the observed differences between treated and control subjects cannot be expected to represent the true differences exactly, because of random variation in both of the groups being compared. Statistical tests help make inferences about the true state of affairs. Why not measure the true state of affairs directly and do away with this uncertainty? The reason is that research must ordinarily be conducted on a sample of patients and not all patients with the condition under study. As a result, there is always a possibility that the particular sample of patients in a study, even though selected in an unbiased way, might not be representative of the whole.

In the usual situation, where the principal conclusions of a trial are expressed in dichotomous terms, (i.e., the treatment is considered to be either successful or not) there are four ways in which those conclusions might relate to reality (Fig. 9.1).

Two of the four possibilities lead to correct conclusions: when the treatments really do have different effects, and that is the conclusion of the study; and when the treatments really have similar effects, and the study concludes this is so.

There are also two ways of being wrong. The treatments under study may be actually no better than no treatment, but it is concluded that the study treatment is better. Error of this kind, resulting in a "false positive" conclusion that the treatment is effective, is referred to as α or *Type I* error. Alpha is the error of saying that there is a difference when there is not. On the other hand, treatment might be effective, but the study concludes that it is not. This "false negative" conclusion is called a β or *Type II* error. Beta is the error of saying that there is no difference when there is one. "No difference" is a simplified way of saying that the true

		TRUE DIFFERENCE	
		Present	Absent
CONCLUSION OF STATISTICAL TEST	Different	Correct	Incorrect: Type I (α) Error
	Not Different	Incorrect Type II (β) Error	Correct

Figure 9.1. The relationship between the results of a statistical test and the true difference between two treatment groups. ("Absent" is a simplification. It really means that the true difference is not greater than a specified amount.)

difference is unlikely to be larger than a certain size. It is not possible to establish that there is no difference at all between two treatments.

The reader may recognize that Figure 9.1 is similar to the four-fold table comparing the results of a diagnostic test to the true diagnosis (Chapter 3). Here the "test" is the conclusion of a clinical trial, based on a statistical test of results from a sample of patients. Reality is the true relative merits of the treatments being compared, if they could be established for all patients with the illness under study—for example, by making observations on all patients or a large number of samples of patients. The α error is analogous to a false positive and β error to a false negative test result. In the absence of bias, random variation is responsible for the uncertainty of the statistical conclusion.

Because random variation plays a part in all observations, it is an oversimplification to ask whether or not chance accounted for the results. Rather, it is a question of how likely random variation is to have determined the findings under the particular conditions of the study. The probability of error due to random variation is estimated by means of *inferential statistics*, a quantitative science that, based on assumptions about the mathematical properties of the data, allows calculations of the probability that the results could have occurred by chance alone.

Statistics is a specialized field with its own jargon—variance, regression, universe, power—that is unfamiliar to many clinicians. However, leaving aside the genuine complexity of statistical method, inferential statistics should be regarded by the nonexpert as a useful means to an end. Statistical tests are the means by which the effects of random variation are estimated.

The next two sections will discuss α and β error, respectively. We will attempt to place inferential statistics, as they are used to estimate the probabilities of these errors, in context. However, we will make no attempt to deal with these subjects in a rigorous, quantitative fashion. For that, the reader is referred to a number of excellent textbooks of biostatistics (see Suggested Readings.)

CONCLUDING THAT A TREATMENT WORKS

Most of the inferential statistics encountered in the current medical literature concern the likelihood of an α error and are expressed by the familiar *p value*. The p value is a quantitative statement of the probability that observed differences in the particular study at hand could have happened by chance alone, assuming that there is in fact no difference between the groups in the long run. Another way of expressing this is that p is an answer to the question: If there were no difference between treatments and the trial was repeated many times, what proportion of the trials would lead to the conclusion that a treatment is effective?

We will call the p value "p_α" to distinguish it from estimates of the other kind of error due to random variation, β error, which we will refer to as p_β. When a simple "p" is found in the scientific literature it ordinarily refers to what we have called p_α. The kind of error estimated by p_α applies whenever it is concluded that one treatment is more effective than another. If it is concluded that there is no difference between treatments, then p_α is not relevant; in that situation, p_β (probability of β error) applies.

It has become customary to attach special significance to p values falling below 0.05. This is because it is generally agreed that one chance in twenty is a small risk of being wrong. One in twenty is so small, in fact, that it is reasonable to conclude that such an occurrence is unlikely to have arisen by chance alone. It could have arisen by chance, and one in twenty times it will. But it is unlikely.

Differences associated with p_α less than 0.05 are called "statistically significant." It is important to remember, however, that setting a cut-off point at 0.05 is entirely arbitrary. Reasonable people might accept higher values or insist on lower ones, depending on the consequences of a false positive conclusion in a given situation.

To accommodate various opinions about what is and is not unlikely, some researchers report the actual probabilities of an α error (e.g., 0.03, 0.07, 0.11, etc.), rather than lumping them into two categories, <0.05 or ≥0.05. The interpretation of what is statistically significant is then left to the reader. However, p values greater than one in five are usually reported as simply $p_\alpha > 0.20$ because nearly everyone can agree that a probability of an α error that is greater than one in five is an unacceptably high risk.

Statistical Significance and Clinical Importance

A statistically significant difference, no matter how small the p_α, does not mean that the difference is clinically important. For example, a p value of $p < 0.0001$, if it emerged from a well-designed study, conveys a high degree of confidence that a difference really exists. But this p_α tells us nothing about the magnitude of that difference or its clinical importance. In fact, entirely trivial differences may be highly statistically significant if a large enough number of patients are studied.

Example—Dietary calcium is negatively associated with hypertension in surveys of adult Americans. McCarron et al. conducted a randomized, double-blind, placebo-controlled trial to see if supplemental calcium reduces blood pressure (2). Forty-eight patients with hypertension were given either 1000 mg/day of oral calcium or placebo. After 8 weeks, blood pressure (supine) was reduced in the calcium-treated group by 5.6 mm Hg systolic and 2.3 mm Hg diastolic pressure (both $p < .05$).

The existence of this reduction, established by a strong research design and low p value, may be an important clue in efforts to understand the biology of hypertension. However, the magnitude of the reduction is not large enough to make dietary calcium supplementation a particularly useful way of treating clinical hypertension.

On the other hand, very unimpressive p_α values can result from studies showing strong treatment effects if there are few subjects in the study (see the following section).

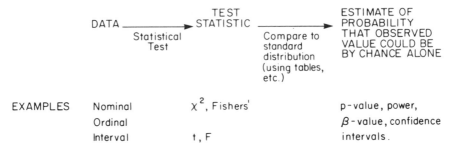

Figure 9.2. Statistical tests.

Statistical Tests

Basic statistical tests, familiar to many readers, are used to estimate the probability of an α error. A summary of commonly used statistical tests and the kinds of data for which they are used is presented in Figure 9.2. The validity of each test depends on certain assumptions about the data. If the data at hand do not satisfy these assumptions, the resulting p_α may be misleading. A discussion of how these statistical tests are derived and calculated and of the assumptions upon which they rest can be found in a number of excellent textbooks of biostatistics.

Statistics are also used to describe the degree of association between variables. Familiar expressions of association are Pearson's product moment correlation (r) for interval data and Spearman's rank correlation for ordinal data. Each of these statistics expresses in quantitative terms the extent to which the value of one variable is associated with the value of a second variable. Each has a corresponding statistical test to assess whether the observed association is greater than might have arisen by chance alone.

One- and Two-Tailed Tests

For a given set of data, the p values obtained depend on whether it is assumed from the outset that meaningful differences could only occur in one direction. For example, it might be generally believed that a relatively innocuous treatment could only help and could not do harm. If we are prepared to make this assumption, then statistical tests can be conducted in such a way that a given difference favoring treatment is more likely to be statistically significant than if we are not. When the possibility of a difference in either direction is entertained, a *two-tailed* test of significance is used, whereas if we consider only differences in a particular direction, a *one-tailed* test is used. These terms come from the appearance of a curve describing the random variation in differences between treatments of equal value, where the two tails of the curve include statistically unlikely sample results favoring one or the other treatment (Fig. 9.3).

There are differences of opinion about which approach—one- or two-tailed—is most appropriate in general, and for specific studies as well. Two-tailed tests are more conservative; they are less likely to conclude that a treatment works when it does not, but run a greater risk of missing a

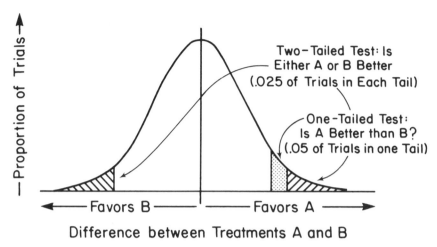

Figure 9.3. One- and two-tailed tests of statistical significance, where $p_\alpha = 0.05$. A larger observed difference in favor of treatment is required for statistical significance if the analysis is done assuming that either *A* or *B* might be better.

true difference favoring treatment. On the other hand, one-tailed tests assume that one of the treatments is not worse, an assumption that is not necessarily correct.

CONCLUDING THAT A TREATMENT DOES NOT WORK

Some trials come to the conclusion that a new treatment is no better than the old. There are some very influential examples: studies showing that coronary artery bypass surgery does not prolong life in patients with chronic stable angina (except for those with left main coronary artery obstruction); the failure of insulin, as compared to diet alone, to reduce complication rates in patients with mild diabetes mellitus; and the failure of extracranial/intracranial bypass surgery to prevent strokes.

The question arises: Could results like these have occurred by chance alone? Could the findings of such trials have misrepresented the truth because these particular studies had the bad luck to turn out in relatively unlikely ways? Specifically, what is the probability of a false negative study: a β or Type II error expressed as p_β? The risk of a false negative study is particularly large in small studies.

Until recently, it has been unusual to find a careful consideration of p_β when the results of clinical trials were presented. Why have "negative trials" so rarely been subjected to the appropriate statistical testing in published research? One reason is that the mathematical basis of p_β is more difficult to conceptualize than p_α. Beta is relatively tough going for beginners. As a result, nearly all the space in introductory textbooks is devoted to p_α and usually only a few pages are given to p_β. Because most of us never get beyond introductory statistics, if that, we have very little exposure to the possibility of β error.

It may also be that β is neglected because we all simply prefer things that work. Negative results are unwelcome for most studies. If negative studies are reported at all, the authors may prefer to emphasize subgroups of patients in which treatment differences are found, even if the differences are not statistically significant. Authors may also focus on reasons other than chance that explain why true differences might have been missed.

Whatever the reason for not considering the probability of β error, it is the main question that should be asked when the results of a study indicate "no difference." Often the risk of β error is surprisingly large. In a survey of 71 published controlled trials showing no therapeutic benefit, 67 had a greater than 10% risk of missing a true therapeutic improvement of 25% (3). Fifty of the 71 trials had at least a 10% risk of missing a 50% improvement. The authors commented that "either these trials were almost uniformly undersized in the planning stage or the expected reduction in the end point percentage due to the treatment under consideration was very much in excess of a 50% reduction, and the reduction did not take place."

The probability that a trial will find a statistically significant difference when a difference really exists is called *statistical power*.

$$\text{Statistical Power} = 1 - p_\beta$$

Power and p_β are complementary ways of expressing the same concept. Power is analogous to the sensitivity of a diagnostic test. In fact, one speaks of a study being powerful if it has a high probability of detecting as different all those treatments that really are different.

How Many Patients are Enough

Suppose you are reading about a clinical trial comparing a promising new therapy to the current form of treatment. You are aware that random variation can be the source of whatever differences are observed, and you wonder if the number of patients (*sample size*) in this study is large enough to make chance an unlikely explanation for what was found. How many patients would be necessary to make an adequate comparison of the effects of the two treatments? The answer depends on four characteristics of the study: the difference in outcome between treatment groups, p_α, p_β and the nature of the data being studied. Each is described below.

- **Effect size**
  Sample size depends on the magnitude of the difference to be detected. We are free to look for differences of any magnitude, and of course, we hope to be able to detect even very small differences. But more patients are needed to detect small differences, everything else being equal. So it is best to ask only that there is a sufficient number of patients to detect the degree of improvement that would be clinically meaningful. On the other hand, if we are interested in detecting only very large differences between treated and control groups (i.e., strong treatment effects), then fewer patients need be studied.

- **Alpha error**

Sample size is also related to the risk of an alpha error: concluding that treatment is effective when it is not. The acceptable size for a risk of this kind is a value judgment. There are no theoretical limits as to how large or small that risk must be (short of 0 and 1). If one is prepared to accept the consequences of a large chance of falsely concluding that the therapy is valuable, one can reach conclusions with relatively few patients. On the other hand, if one wants to take only a small risk of being wrong in this way, a larger number of patients will be required. As we discussed earlier, it is customary to set p_α at 0.05 (1 in 20) or sometimes 0.01.

- **Beta error**

The chosen risk of a β error is another determinant of sample size. An acceptable probability of this error is also a judgment that can be freely made and changed, to suit individual tastes. P_β is often set at 0.20, a 20% chance of missing true differences in a particular study of a given size.

- **Characteristics of the data**

The statistical power of a study is also determined by the nature of the data. When the outcome is expressed on a nominal scale and so is described by counts or proportions of events, its statistical power depends on the rate of events: The larger the rate of events, the greater the statistical power for a given number of people at risk. As Peto et al. put it,

> In clinical trials of time to death (or of the time to some other particular "event"—relapse, metastasis, first thrombosis, stroke, recurrence, or time to death from a particular cause), the ability of the trial to distinguish between the merits of two treatments depends on how many patients die (or suffer a relevant event), rather than on the number of patients entered. A study of 100 patients, 50 of whom die, is about as sensitive as a study with 1000 patients, 50 of whom die (4).

If the outcome is a continuous variable, such as blood pressure or serum cholesterol, power is affected by the degree to which patients vary among themselves: The greater the variation from patient to patient with respect to the characteristic being measured, the more difficult it is to be confident that the observed differences (or lack of difference) between groups is not because of this variation, rather than true difference between the treatment effects. In other words, the larger the variation among patients, the lower the statistical power.

In designing a study, the investigator chooses the size of treatment effect and the Type I and Type II errors he or she will accept. But an investigator cannot control the way that the characteristics of the data determine statistical power.

Interrelationships

The interrelationships among these four variables are summarized in Table 9.1. The variables in Table 9.1 can be traded off against each other. In general, for any given number of subjects there is a trade-off between α

Table 9.1

Determinants of Sample Size

	DETERMINED BY		
	INVESTIGATOR		THE DATA
N varies according to	$\dfrac{1}{\Delta, P_\alpha, P_\beta}$	and	$\dfrac{V}{I}$ or $\dfrac{I}{P}$

N = Number of patients studied
Δ = Size of difference in outcome between groups
P_α = Probability of an a (Type I) error, i.e., false positive results
P_β = Probability of a b (Type II) error, i.e., false negative result
V = Variability of observations (for interval data)
P = Proportion of patients experiencing outcome of interest (for nominal data)

and β error. Everything else being equal, the more one is willing to accept one kind of error, the less it will be necessary to risk the other. Neither kind of error is inherently worse than the other. The consequences of using erroneous information depend on the clinical situation. When a better treatment is badly needed—for example, when the disease is very dangerous and no satisfactory alternative treatment is available—it would be reasonable to accept a relatively high risk of concluding a new treatment is effective when it really is not (large α error) in order to minimize the possibility of missing a valuable treatment (low β error). On the other hand, if the disease is less serious, alternative treatments are available, or the new treatment is expensive or dangerous, one might want to minimize the risk of accepting the new treatment when it is not really effective (low α error), even at the expense of a relatively large chance of missing an effective treatment (large β error). It is of course possible to reduce both α and β error if the number of patients is increased, outcome events are more frequent, variability is decreased, or a larger treatment effect is sought.

For conventional levels of p_α and p_β the effect of the strength of treatment on the number of subjects is illustrated by the following examples, one representing a situation in which a very large number of patients was required and the other in which a relatively small number of patients was sufficient.

Example (Large sample size)—The British Medical Research Council conducted a randomized controlled trial to determine whether drug treatment of mild hypertension (phase V diastolic blood pressure 90–109 mm Hg) reduced the rate of stroke, of death due to hypertension, and of coronary events in men and women aged 35–64 years. The investigators knew from the beginning that both the rate of outcome events and the treatment effect would be relatively small, so that a large number of patients had to be entered in the trial. In the planning phase, it was estimated that 18,000 people would have to be followed for 5 years (90,000 person-years of observation) in order to detect a 40% reduction in the number of deaths due to strokes, with an alpha error of 1% and a beta error of 5%. They also expected that there would be large enough numbers of fatal and nonfatal coronary events to assess treatment for these outcomes.

When the study was completed, 17,354 people had been observed for 85,572 person-years. There was a 46% reduction in stroke rate ($p < .01$) and an 18% reduction in all cardiovascular events ($p < .05$) in the treated group, but no difference in overall rate of coronary events or mortality from all causes (5).

Example (Small sample size)—To evaluate the efficacy of cimetidine in severe duodenal ulceration, 40 patients with active duodenal ulcers seen on endoscopy were randomly allocated to receive cimetidine (1 gm/day) or placebo. After 4 weeks, a second endoscopy was performed by physicians who did not know which treatment had been given. Ulcer healing was observed in 17 of 20 patients receiving cimetidine and 5 of 20 patients receiving placebo. This difference was highly statistically significant ($p < 0.0005$) (6).

In this trial, the treatment effect was so powerful that relatively few patients were needed to establish it.

For most of the therapeutic questions we encounter today, a surprisingly large number of patients are required. The value of dramatic, powerful treatments, such as insulin for diabetic ketoacidosis, could be established with a small number of subjects. But such treatments come along rarely, and many of them are already well established. We are left with diseases, many of them chronic, for which advances are usually modest and come about through small increments. This places special importance on whether the size of clinical trials is adequate to distinguish real from chance effects.

Clinicians should develop some facility for estimating the power of published studies. Toward that end, Figure 9.4 shows the relationship between sample size and treatment difference for several baseline rates for outcome events. It is apparent from Figure 9.4 that studies involving fewer than 100 patients have a rather poor chance of detecting statistically significant differences of even large treatment effects. Also, it is difficult to detect effect sizes of less than 25%.

In practice, statistical power can be estimated by means of readily available formulas, tables, nomograms, or computer programs.

Statistical Power After a Study is Completed

The statistical power that a study actually has, after it has been completed, is different from the power that was estimated in advance (7). This is because there is more information. There are point estimates of rates in the two groups being compared and estimates of the variability in their responses. For example, if the results show a trend favoring the placebo group, it is much less likely that the experimental treatment is actually better, as compared to the situation where the experimental group had fared better, but the results fell just short of statistical significance.

Detecting Rare Events

Often it is important to detect a relatively uncommon event—for example, 1/1000—particularly if that event is severe, such as aplastic

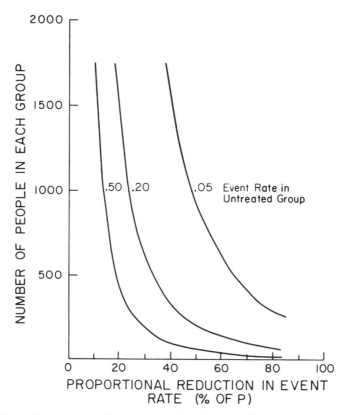

Figure 9.4. The number of people required in each of two treatment groups (of equal size) to have an 80% chance of detecting a difference (p = .05) in a given outcome rate between treated and untreated patients, for various rates (*P*) of outcome events in the untreated group. (Calculated from formula in Weiss NS: *Clinical Epidemiology. The study of the outcome of illness.* New York, Oxford University Press, 1986.)

anemia or life-threatening arrhythmia following drug intake. In such cases, a great many people must be observed in order to detect even one such event, much less to develop a relatively stable estimate of its frequency.

Figure 9.5 shows for several rates the probability of detecting an event as a function of the number of people under observation. A rule of thumb is: In order to have a good chance of detecting a 1/x event one needs to observe 3x people (8). For example, to detect a 1/1000 event, one would need to observe 3000 people.

POINT ESTIMATES AND CONFIDENCE INTERVALS

The exact effect size—for example, treatment effect in a clinical trial— observed in a particular study is called the *point estimate* of effect. It is the

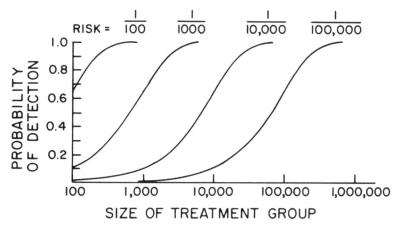

Figure 9.5. The probability of detecting one event according to the rate of the event and the number of people observed. (From Guess HA, Rudnick SA: Use of cost-effectiveness analysis in planning cancer chemoprophylaxis trials. *Controlled Clin Trials* 4:89–100, 1983.)

best estimate from the study of the true effect size and is the summary statistic usually given the most emphasis in reports of research.

The statistical precision (stability of the estimate) of an observed effect size increases with the statistical power of the study. This precision is often expressed as a *confidence interval*, usually the 95% confidence interval, around the point estimate. Confidence intervals around an effect size are interpreted as: If the study is unbiased, there is a 95% chance that the interval includes the true effect size. The narrower the confidence interval, the more certain one can be about the size of the true effect. To be more specific, the true value is most likely to be close to the point estimate, less likely to be near the outer limits of the interval, and could (5 times out of 100) fall outside these limits altogether.

Confidence intervals are an alternative way of expressing statistical significance. If the value corresponding to no effect falls outside 95% confidence intervals, the results are statistically significant at the .05 level; if the confidence intervals include this point, the results are not statistically significant.

Confidence intervals also provide information about statistical power. If the confidence interval barely includes the value corresponding to no effect and is relatively wide, a significant difference might have been found if the study had had more power.

Example—Figure 9.6 illustrates point estimates and confidence intervals for the estimated relative risk of exogenous estrogens for three diseases: endometrial cancer, myocardial infarction, and hip fracture. (Notice that the risk is on a log scale, giving the superficial impression that confidence intervals for the higher risks are narrower than they really are.)

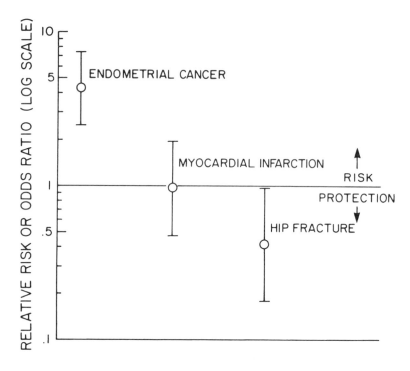

Figure 9.6. Point estimates (*O*) and confidence intervals (*I*): the risks and benefits of exogenous estrogens for postmenopausal women. (Data from Antunes CM, Stolley PD, Rosenshein NB, Davies JL et al: Endometrial cancer and estrogen use. Report of a large case control study. *N Engl J Med* 300:9–13, 1979; Rosenberg L, Armstrong B, Jick H: Myocardial infarction and estrogen therapy in post-menopausal women. *N Engl J Med* 294:1256–1259, 1976; and Paganini-Hill A, Ross RK, Gerkins VR, Henderson BE, Arthur M, Mack TM: Menopausal estrogen therapy and hip fractures. *Ann Intern Med* 95:28–31, 1981.)

The best estimate of risk for endometrial cancer is 4.3, but the true value is not precisely estimated and could easily be as high as 7.5 or as low as 1.5. In any case, it is unlikely to be as low as 1.0 (no risk).

In contrast, based on the data presented estrogens are unlikely to be a risk factor for myocardial infarction; the best estimate is no risk, although the data are consistent with either a very small harmful or a small protective effect.

Finally, estrogens are likely to protect against hip fracture. That the upper boundary of the confidence interval falls below 1.0 is another way of indicating that the protective effect is statistically significant at the .05 level.

Point estimates and confidence intervals are used to characterize the statistical precision of any rate (incidence, prevalence), comparisons of rates (relative and attributable risk), or other summary statistics.

MULTIPLE COMPARISONS

The statistical conclusions of research have an aura of authority that defies challenge, particularly by nonexperts. But as many skeptics have suspected, it is possible to "lie with statistics," even if unintentionally. What is more, this is possible even if the research is well designed, the mathematics flawless, and the investigators' intentions beyond reproach.

Statistical conclusions can be misleading because the strength of statistical tests depends on the number of research questions considered in the study and when those questions were asked. If many comparisons are made among the variables in a large set of data, the p value associated with each individual comparison is an underestimate of how often the result of that comparison, among the others, is likely to arise by chance. As implausible as it might seem, the interpretation of the p value from a single statistical test depends on the context in which it is done.

To understand how this might happen, consider the following example. Suppose a large study has been done in which there are multiple subgroups of patients and many different outcomes. For example, it might be a clinical trial of the value of a treatment for coronary artery disease, where patients fall into several clinically meaningful groups (e.g., 1, 2, and 3-vessel disease, good and bad ventricular function, the presence or absence of arrhythmias, and various combinations of these) and several outcomes are considered, e.g., death, myocardial infarction, angina, etc. Suppose also that there are no true associations between treatment and outcome for any of the subgroups and any of the outcomes. Finally, suppose that the effects of treatment are assessed separately for each subgroup and for each outcome—a process that involves a great many comparisons. As pointed out earlier in this chapter, at p = 0.05, one in 20 of these comparisons is likely to be "statistically significant." If 40 comparisons are made, on the average, 2 would be found to be statistically significant; if 100 comparisons are made, about 5 would be likely to emerge as "significant;" and so on. When a great many comparisons have been made, there is a chance that a few will be found that are unusual enough, because of random variation, that they exceed the level of statistical significance even though no true associations between variables exist in nature. The more comparisons that are made, the more likely that one of them will be found statistically significant.

The situation we have just described is referred to as the *multiple comparisons* problem. Because of this problem, the strength of evidence from clinical research depends on how focused its questions were at the outset.

Unfortunately, when the results of research are presented, it is not always possible to know how many comparisons were really made. Often, interesting findings are selected from a larger number of uninteresting ones. This process of deciding what is and is not important about a mass of data can introduce considerable distortion of reality.

How can the statistical effects of multiple comparisons be taken into account when interpreting research? Although a variety of ways of adjusting p_α have been proposed, for the present the best advice is to be aware of the problem and to be cautious about accepting positive conclusions of studies where multiple comparisons were made. As one statistician put it:

> If you dredge the data sufficiently deep and sufficiently often, you will find something odd. Many of these bizarre findings will be due to chance. I do not imply that data dredging is not an occupation for honorable persons, but rather that discoveries that were not initially postulated as among the major objectives of the trial should be treated with extreme caution. Statistical theory may in due course show us how to allow for such incidental findings. At present, I think the best attitude to adopt is caution, coupled with an attempt to confirm or refute the findings by further studies (9).

There are several ways of dealing with this problem, which will be discussed in Chapter 12.

SUMMARY

Clinical information is based on observations made on samples of patients. Yet, even unbiased samples may misrepresent events in a larger population of such patients, because of the effects of random variation among its members.

Inferential statistics are used to estimate the role of random variation in clinical observations. When two treatments are compared, there are two ways in which the conclusions of the trial can be wrong: The treatments may be no different and it is concluded one is better; or one treatment may be better, and it is concluded there is no difference. The probabilities that these errors will occur in a given situation are called p_α and p_β, respectively.

The power of a statistical test $(1 - p_\beta)$ is the probability of finding a statistically significant difference when a difference of a given size really exists. Statistical power is related to the number of patients in the trial, size of the treatment effect, p_α, and the rate of outcome events or variability of responses among patients. Everything else being equal, power can be increased by increasing the number of patients in a trial, but that is not always feasible.

Individual studies run an increased risk of reporting a false positive result if many subsets of the data are compared; they are at increased risk of a false negative result if they lack statistical power, usually because they include too few patients or outcome events are uncommon.

REFERENCES

1. Johnson AF: Beneath the technological fix. Outliers and probability statements. *J Chron Dis* 38:957–961, 1985.
2. McCarron DA, Morris CD: Blood pressure response to oral calcium in persons with mild to moderate hypertension. *Ann Intern Med* 103:825–831, 1985.
3. Freiman JA, Chalmers TC, Smith H Jr, Kuebler RR: The importance of beta, the type

II error and sample size in the design and interpretation of the randomized control trial. *N Engl J Med* 299:690–694, 1978.

4. Peto R, Pike MC, Armitage P, Breslow NE, Cox DR, Howard SV, Mantel N, McPherson K, Peto J, Smith PG: Design and analysis of randomized clinical trials requiring prolonged observation of each patient. I. Introduction and design. *Br J Cancer* 34:585–612, 1976.
5. Medical Research Council Working Party: MRC trial of treatment of mild hypertension; principal results. *Br Med J* 291:97–104, 1985.
6. Gray GR, McKenzie I, Smith IS, Crean GP, Gillespie G: Oral cimetidine in severe duodenal ulceration. A double-blind controlled trial. *Lancet* 1:4–7, 1977.
7. Detsky AS, Sackett DL: When is a "negative" clinical trial big enough? How many patients you need depends on what you found. *Arch Intern Med* 145:709–712, 1985.
8. Sackett, DL, Haynes RB, Gent M, Taylor DW: Compliance. In Inman WHW (ed): *Monitoring for Drug Safety.* Lancaster, UK, MTP Press, 1980.
9. Armitage P. Importance of prognostic factors in the analysis of data from clinical trials. *Controlled Clin Trials* 1:347–353, 1981.

SUGGESTED READINGS

Abt K: Problems of repeated significance testing. *Controlled Clin Trials* 1:377–381, 1981.

Altman DG, Gore SM, Gardner MJ, Pocock SJ: Statistical guidelines for contributors to medical journals. *Br Med J* 286:1489–1493, 1983.

Bailar JC III, Mosteller F, Editors. *Medical Uses of Statistics.* Waltham, Massachusetts, NEJM Books, 1986.

Berwick DM: Experimental power: the other side of the coin. *Pediatrics* 65:1043–1045, 1980.

Cupples LA, Heeren T, Schatzkin A, Colton T: Multiple testing of hypotheses in comparing two groups. *Ann Intern Med* 100:122–129, 1984.

Detsky AS, Sackett DL: When was a "negative" clinical trial big enough? How many patients you need depends on what you found. *Arch Intern Med* 145:709–712, 1985.

Feinstein AR: *Clinical Biostatistics.* Section 4. Mathematical Mistiques and Statistical Strategies. St. Louis, C V Mosby, 1977.

Feinstein AR: *Clinical Epidemiology. The Architecture of Clinical Research. Part 2: Outline of Statistical Strategies.* Philadelphia, W B Saunders, 1985.

Freiman JA, Chalmers TC, Smith H Jr, Kuebler RR: The importance of beta, the type II error and sample size in the design and interpretation of the randomized control trial. *N Engl J Med* 299:690–694, 1978.

Ingelfinger JA, Mosteller F, Thibodeau LA, Ware JH: *Biostatistics in Clinical Medicine.* New York, MacMillan, 1983.

Lew RA, Day CL Jr, Harrist TJ, Wood WC, Mihm MC: Multivariate analysis. Some guidelines for physicians. *JAMA* 249:641–643, 1983.

Moses LE: Statistical concepts fundamental to investigations. *N Engl J Med* 312:890–897, 1985.

Rothman KJ: A show of confidence. *N Engl J Med* 299:1362–1363, 1978.

Swinscow, TDV: *Statistics at Square One* ed 4. London, British Medical Association, 1978.

Tukey JW: Some thoughts on clinical trials, especially problems of multiplicity. *Science* 198:679–684, 1977.

Young MJ, Bresnitz EA, Strom BL: Sample size nomograms for interpreting negative clinical studies. *Ann Intern Med* 99:248–251, 1983.

chapter 10

RARE DISEASE

It has been estimated that 90% of medical school curriculum time considers 10% of mankind's morbidity. This estimate has been used to derogate the emphasis placed by academic centers on rare diseases. But it also highlights an inescapable fact—most diseases are, thankfully, not common. For example, the current epidemic of lung cancer has been called the "plague of the 20th century." However, the bubonic plague killed in a matter of months as many as 60–70% of the residents of afflicted cities and villages in 14th-century Europe. Lung cancer, on the other hand, will kill approximately 3–4% of older men over a 10-year period. Although certainly a tragic and largely preventable disease, this "common" killer will be diagnosed only once a year or less by the average primary care physician. To put this frequency into the perspective of a cohort study, 3000 older men must be followed for at least 10 years in order to obtain information about 100 cases.

What about the prevalence of the common chronic diseases? After all, prevalence provides a better estimate of the physician's caseload than incidence. Asthma, generally considered a relatively common disease, was reported by 3% of a random sample of Americans. However, the large majority of these people (80% or more) suffered no disability related to their asthma, and 30% did not visit a physician for any reason during a 1-year period (1). Based on these figures, it has been estimated that the identification of 200 asthmatics under age 55 would require a survey of 2300 households or the review of 10,700 medical records from primary care practices (2).

The difficulties attending the acquisition of large numbers of patients with an uncommon condition forces investigators and clinicians to confine their observations of many diseases to relatively small numbers of people. The question is whether studies of small numbers of patients are useful to the practitioner facing problems of diagnosis, prognosis, cause, or treatment, given all the pitfalls described in the preceding chapters. Or, to turn the question around a little, under what circumstances can observations on small numbers of patients prove useful?

STUDIES OF FEW PATIENTS

Case Reports

Case reports are detailed presentations of a single case or a handful of cases. They represent an important way in which unusual diseases or unusual presentations of disease are brought to the attention of the medical community. A systematic review of the original articles published in the *Journal of the American Medical Association, The Lancet,* and the *New England Journal of Medicine* in the years 1946, 1956, 1966, and 1976 revealed that 38% of all research reports in these prestigious journals studied ten or fewer subjects and 13% discussed a single case (3). Reports of rare events, therefore, are not rare.

Case reports serve several different purposes. First, they are virtually our only means of surveillance for rare clinical events. Therefore, they are a rich source of ideas (hypotheses) about disease frequency, risk, prognosis, and treatment. Case reports rarely can be used to test these hypotheses, but they do place issues before the medical community and often trigger more decisive studies. Some conditions that were first recognized through case reports include birth defects from thalidomide, the fetal alcohol syndrome, and some of the legionella infections.

Case reports also serve to elucidate the mechanisms of disease and treatment by reporting highly detailed and methodologically sophisticated clinical and laboratory studies of a patient or small group of patients. In this instance, the complexity, cost, and the often experimental nature of the investigations limit their application to small numbers of patients. Such studies have contributed a great deal to our understanding of the genetic, metabolic, and physiologic basis of a large number of human diseases. These studies represent the bridge between laboratory research and clinical research and have a well-established place in the annals of medical progress.

The following is an example of how a report of a single case can reveal a great deal about the mechanism of a disease.

Example—The anesthetic halothane has been suspected of causing hepatitis. However, because the frequency of hepatitis after exposure to halothane is low and there are many other causes of hepatitis after surgery, "halothane hepatitis" has been controversial.

Experience with a single individual helped clarify the problem (4). An anesthetist was found to have recurrent hepatitis, leading to cirrhosis. Attacks of hepatitis regularly recurred within hours of his return to work. When he was exposed to small doses of halothane under experimental conditions, his hepatitis recurred and was well documented by clinical observations, biochemical tests, and liver histology.

Because of this unusual case, it is clear that halothane can cause hepatitis. But the case report provides no information on how often this occurs.

Another use of the case report is to present unusual manifestations of disease. Sometimes this can become the medical version of Ripley's *Believe It or Not*, an informal compendium of medical oddities where the interest lies in the sheer unbelievability of the case. The larger the lesion and the more outrageous the foreign body or its location, the more likely a case report is to find its way into the literature. Oddities that are simply bizarre aberrations from the usual course of events may titillate, but reveal little of clinical importance.

Some so-called oddities are, however, the result of a fresher, more insightful look at a problem and prove to be the first evidence of a subsequently useful finding. The problem for the reader is how to distinguish between the freak and the fresh insight. There are no rules of which we are aware. When all else fails, one can only rely on common sense and a well-developed sense of skepticism.

Because case reports involve a small and highly selected group of patients, they are particularly susceptible to bias. For example, case reports of successful therapy may be misleading because journals are unlikely to receive or publish case reports of unsuccessful therapy. Dietz compared reports of the effectiveness of postmortem cesarean section in an attempt to save the baby in 105 instances found in 63 case reports and 72 instances reported from a single community-based study (5). The contrast in findings was striking; whereas 57% of the infants described in case reports survived, only 15% of infants in the community-based study survived. The obvious explanation rests with the tendency of authors to write up and journal editors to accept for publication the unusual; in this example, those cases with an unusually happy ending. At the other extreme, disasters written up in case reports often prove, on more systematic study of larger populations, to be rare phenomena.

Perhaps the wisest stance to take when reviewing a case report is to use it as a signal to look for further evidence of the described phenomenon in the literature or among your patients. With very few exceptions, case reports should not serve as the basis for altering clinical practice because of their inherent biases and their inability to estimate the frequency of the described occurrence or the role of chance.

The Joint Occurrence of Rare Events

Case reports often describe the joint occurrence of uncommon events, particularly if the observed association lends itself to an interesting biologic explanation. But even rare events occur together by chance alone; simply observing this occurrence does not mean they are biologically related. As one author put it, "In a large population the issue is not whether rare events occur, but whether they occur more frequently than expected by chance (6)."

Table 10.1 illustrates how often two uncommon conditions, end-stage

Table 10.1

The Joint Occurrence of Two Rare Conditions: An Estimate of the Frequency and Number of Cases of Exposure to a Nonsteroidal Anti-Inflammatory Drug and End-Stage Renal Failure Occurring Together if the Two were not Biologically Related

Frequency separately	
Prevalence of use of the drug (hypothetical)	1/100 persons
Incidence of end-stage renal disease	40/1,000,000/year
Incidence of joint occurrence	1/100 × 40/1,000,000/year
	= 4/10,000,000/year
Population of North America	250,000,000
Cases in North America	4/10,000,000/Year × 250,000,000
	= 100/year

[a] Data on incidence of renal failure from Hiatt RA, Friedman GD: Characteristics of patients referred for treatment of end-stage renal disease in a defined population. *Am J Public Health* 72: 829–833, 1982.

renal failure and use of a specific nonsteroidal antiinflammatory drug, might occur together by chance alone. If there were no biologic association between the two, then the probability that they would occur together is the product of their separate frequencies. In North America alone, 100 cases would occur—more than enough to spawn several case reports.

There are also reasons why such cases might be seen in medical centers and be reported in the literature out of proportion to their frequency in the population at large. Patients with two severe diseases might be more likely to be admitted to hospitals than if they had either alone, simply because they are sicker. It has also been shown that two diseases not associated in the general population can be associated in hospitals if patients with the two diseases are admitted at different rates (7). Moreover, patients with two diseases are more interesting and so are more likely to be written up in articles that are submitted to journals and accepted for publication.

Therefore, one should be skeptical about reports of associations that are based on case reports only. They are simply hypotheses to be tested by stronger methods before being believed.

Case Series

A *case series* is a prevalence survey of a group of individuals with a particular disease, performed at a single point in time. It is a particularly common way of delineating the clinical picture of a rare disease and serves this purpose well—but with some important limitations.

First, case series describe, in quantitative terms, the clinical manifestations of disease, both purported causes and effects, at one point in time. They must be distinguished, therefore, from prognostic studies or uncontrolled trials of treatment where a cohort of patients with a disease is followed over time looking for the outcomes of the disease. Case series do not have a time dimension and that restricts their value as a means of studying cause-effect relationships.

Case series also suffer from the absence of a comparison group. As a result, it is difficult to put observed associations in context.

Example—Between June 1981 and February 1983, a few years after AIDS was first recognized and while its manifestations were being defined, researchers from the Center for Disease Control gathered information on 1000 patients living in the United States who met a surveillance definition for the disease. They described demographic/behavioral characteristics of patients and complications of the disease.

Pneumocystis carinii (PCP) was found in 49.7%, Kaposi's sarcoma in 28.4%, and both in 8.3% of patients; 13.6% had opportunistic infections other than PCP. All but 6.1% of the patients could be classified into one or more of the following groups: homosexual or bisexual men, intravenous drug abusers, Haitian natives, or patients with hemophilia.

This report is cross-sectional and includes no comparison group of people without AIDS. Also, the definition of cases excluded some patients who have AIDS by later standards. Nevertheless, because the complications are so uncommon in otherwise well people and the pattern of at-risk groups so striking, the report clarified our view of AIDS and set the stage for more detailed studies of its manifestations and risk factors (8).

CASE CONTROL STUDIES

To find out whether exposure to X is associated with developing disease Y, one needs a study with several features. First, there must be a comparison group that does not have the disease. Second there must be enough people in the study so that chance does not play a large part in the observed results. Third, the groups must be comparable except for the factor of interest. Finally, if one wants to show that an associated factor is a cause, it is necessary to control for all other important differences, other than the exposure of interest, that remain.

Case reports and case series cannot take us this far. Neither can cohort studies, in many situations, because it is impossible to gather enough cases. But there is a solution.

Studies that compare the frequency of a purported risk factor in a group of cases and a group of controls are called *case control studies*. Another name for this kind of study, now outdated, is *retrospective studies*.

The basic design of a case control study is diagrammed in Figure 10.1. Patients who have the disease and a group of otherwise similar people who do not have the disease are selected. The researchers then look backward in time to determine the frequency of exposure in the two groups. These data can be used to estimate the relative risk of disease related to exposure.

Example—Does use of exogenous estrogens after menopause increase the risk of endometrial cancer? Several groups of researchers have addressed this question, using case control studies. How have they gone about it?

First, the researchers must find a group of women suffering from endometrial cancer. For obvious reasons, they would look in hospitals or other cancer treatment

EXPOSURE TO
RISK FACTOR   DISEASE

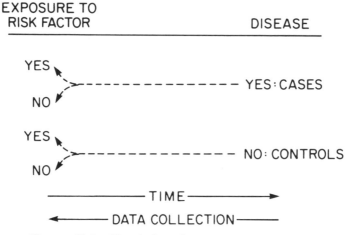

Figure 10.1. The design of case control studies.

centers where many such cases are gathered. The cases, therefore, may not include those who have rapidly succumbed to their disease and would include only women in whom the diagnosis had been made in the course of usual medical care. For example asymptomatic cancer would be unlikely to be included among the cases.

Once the cases are assembled and the diagnosis confirmed, a comparison or *control* group must be selected. Before deciding which people to chose as controls, the investigators must pause to consider the purpose of the study.[a] They want to ascertain whether women with endometrial cancer were more likely to have received estrogen therapy in the past than a similar group of women fortunate enough to have been spared the disease.

What is meant by similar? Similarity in the cohort study would mean membership in the same cohort—for example, postmenopausal women residing in the same community or attending the same clinic. Is there a natural cohort from which a group of cases receiving care at a given hospital can emerge? Because of referral practices, cases assembled at hospitals and other treatment centers usually reside in many communities, receive their care from many physicians, and belong to no common group before becoming ill. Therefore, there is no obviously similar group of women without endometrial cancer and one must be created. This is generally done by finding women who are in the hospital for reasons other than endometrial cancer and/or women residing in the same neighborhoods as the cases. In this way, a group of women is assembled who are, it is hoped, similar to cases with respect to factors that might determine risk for endometrial cancer, other than estrogen use.

Once the cases and controls have been selected and their consent obtained, the

---

[a] For other uses of the word "control," see page 122.

next step is to measure exposure to the risk factor of interest. To examine the possible risk of estrogen therapy, each woman's drug-taking history must be reconstructed for both cases and controls. As opposed to the cohort study, this history will rely on memory and the availability and completeness of medical records. It is the past, not the present, that is important and therein lies a potential for bias in case control studies. As every student of history knows, it is difficult not to interpret the past in the light of one's present condition. For patients, this is particularly so when the present includes a disease as serious as cancer. Investigators can attempt to avoid bias by blinding observers to case status if possible, and by using carefully defined criteria to decide which of the cases and controls received prior estrogen therapy.

The investigators would then estimate the relative risk of estrogen exposure for endometrial cancer, using data on the rates of exposure in cases and controls.

Cohort Versus Case Control Research

Cohort and case control studies are both observational studies of risk factors. Sometimes the two are confused. A distinguishing feature of the case control design is that cases have the outcome of interest at the time that information on risk factors is sought. In cohort research, on the other hand, people are free of disease at the beginning of observation, but are exposed or not exposed to risk factors. Figure 10.2 summarizes how cohort and case control designs differ, using the estrogen/endometrial cancer question as an example.

Case Control Analyses of Prevalence Studies

Cases and controls can be selected in two ways relative to the course of disease. One is to select new (incident) cases—that is, cases of disease as it arises—and controls that were present in the same setting at the same time. The other is to select existing (prevalent) cases from a defined population, as part of a prevalence study. A population is first defined,

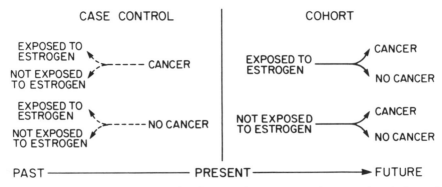

Figure 10.2. A comparison of cohort and case control research: studies of exogenous estrogens as a risk factor for endometrial cancer.

and then at a point in time cases and a much larger number of controls are identified and their exposure is determined.

In general, using incident cases is a stronger way of conducting case control studies. If prevalent cases and controls are used, they can be related to a defined, relatively unselected population, so that there is less opportunity for selection bias. But the disadvantage is that the question addressed by case control studies is ordinarily about incidence: Does exposure to X result in new cases of Y? When prevalent cases are used, the question becomes: Is exposure to X a risk factor for having Y? As discussed in Chapter 4, having Y (prevalence) is determined by both incidence and duration of disease. This problem and its consequences are discussed later in this chapter.

Table 10.2 summarizes the essential characteristics of cohort, case control, and prevalence research designs and illustrates their differences. As will be discussed later, it is these differences that make the case control study particularly susceptible to bias.

The Odds Ratio

How do we decide whether there is an increased risk? Figure 10.3 shows the calculation of risk for cohort and case control studies.

In a cohort study, the susceptible population is divided into two groups— exposed (A + B) and unexposed (C + D)—at the outset. Cases of endometrial cancer emerge naturally over time in the exposed group (A) and the unexposed group (C). This provides us with appropriate numerators and denominators to calculate the incidences of endometrial cancer in the exposed (A/A + B) and unexposed (C/C + D) cohorts. It is also possible to calculate the relative risk.

$$\text{Relative Risk} = \frac{\text{Incidence of Disease in the Exposed}}{\text{Incidence of Disease in the Unexposed}} = \frac{A/A + B}{C/C + D}$$

Case control studies, on the other hand, begin with the selection of a group of cases (A + C) and another group of controls (B + D). There is no way of knowing disease rates because these groups are determined not by nature, but by the investigators' selection criteria. Therefore, an incidence rate of disease among those exposed to estrogen and those not exposed cannot be computed. Consequently, it is not possible to obtain relative risk by dividing incidence among users by incidence among nonusers. What does have meaning, however, are the relative frequencies of women exposed to estrogens among the cases and controls.

It has been demonstrated that one approach for comparing the frequency of exposure among cases and controls provides a measure of risk that is conceptually and mathematically similar to the relative risk. This is the *odds ratio*, defined as the odds[b] that a case is exposed

---

[b] For a reminder of what "odds" means, see page 62.

Table 10.2
Summary of Characteristics of Cohort, Case Control, and Prevalence Designs

	COHORT	CASE CONTROL	PREVALENCE
Population	Begins with a defined population at risk	Population at risk generally undefined	Begins with a defined population
Cases	Cases not selected but ascertained by continuous surveillance (presumably all cases)	Cases selected by investigator from an available pool of patients	Cases not selected but ascertained by a single examination of the population
Controls	Comparison group (i.e., non-cases) not selected—evolve naturally	Controls selected by investigator to resemble cases	Noncases include those free of disease at the single examination
Exposure	Exposure measured before the development of disease	Exposure measured, reconstructed, or recollected after development of disease	Exposure measured, reconstructed, or recollected after development of disease
Measure of Effects	Risk or incidence of disease and relative risk measured directly	Risk or incidence of disease cannot be measured directly: Relative risk of exposure can be estimated by the odds ratio	Risk or incidence of disease cannot be measured directly: Relative risk of exposure can be estimated by the odds ratio

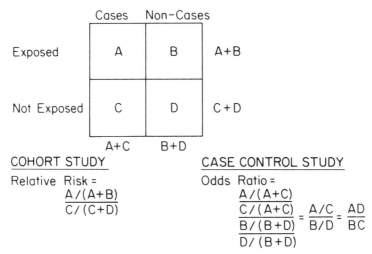

Figure 10.3. Calculation of relative risk for a cohort study and odds ratios (estimated relative risk) for a case control study.

$$\left(\frac{A/A + C}{C/A + C}\right)$$

divided by the odds that a control is exposed

$$\left(\frac{B/B + D}{D/B + D}\right)$$

Under the assumptions discussed below, the odds ratio simplifies to

$$\frac{A/C}{B/D} \text{ or } \frac{A\ D}{B\ C}$$

As is seen in Figure 10.3, the odds ratio can be obtained by multiplying diagonally across the table and then dividing these cross-products.

Note that, if the frequency of exposure is higher among cases, the odds ratio will exceed one, indicating risk. Thus, the stronger the association between the exposure and disease, the higher the odds ratio. Conversely, if the frequency of exposure is lower among cases, the odds ratio will be less than one, indicating protection. The meaning of the odds ratio, therefore, is analogous to the relative risk obtained from cohort studies. The similarity of the information conveyed by the odds ratio and the relative risk has led some investigators to report odds ratios as "estimated relative risks" or simply "relative risks."

The odds ratio is approximately equal to the relative risk only when the incidence of disease is low, because of assumptions that must be made in the calculations. How low must the rates be? The answer depends in part on the size of the relative risk (9). In general, however, distortion of the relative risk becomes large enough to matter at disease rates in unexposed people of greater than about 1/100. Fortunately, most diseases, particularly those examined by means of case control studies, are considerably less common than that rate.

Advantages of Case Control Studies

The case control design is one of the most important methods used to study rare diseases. What are its advantages?

First, the investigators can identify cases unconstrained by the natural frequency of disease and yet can still make a comparison. Cohort studies are quite inefficient for this purpose. For example, in order to gather information about the risk of estrogen use in 100 women with endometrial cancer, one would have to follow a cohort of 10,000 postmenopausal women for about 10 years. Obviously, because of the expense and logistic difficulties of such a study, it would usually not be feasible. In contrast, it has been relatively inexpensive and easy to assemble a hundred or more cases from hospitals and other treatment facilities, find similar groups of women without the disease, and compare frequencies of past estrogen use. In this way, several hundred women can be interviewed in a matter of weeks or months, and an answer can be obtained at a fraction of the cost of a cohort study.

A second advantage of the case control study in exploring the effect of causal or prognostic factors is that one need not wait for a long time for the answer. Many diseases have a long latency—a period of time between exposure to a factor and the expression of its pathologic effects. For example, it has been estimated that 15 or more years may pass before the carcinogenicity of various chemicals becomes manifest. It would require an extremely patient investigator and scientific community to wait for 15 years to see if a suspected risk to health can be confirmed.

Because of their ability to address important questions rapidly and efficiently, case control studies play an increasingly prominent role in the medical literature. If one wants to study cause and effect using a relatively strong method, the case control approach is the only practical way to study some diseases. According to surveys of leading medical journals, case control studies comprise 5–10% of all original articles and 30–40% of all epidemiologic articles (10). Their quickness and cheapness justify their popularity as long as their results are valid; and here is the problem because case control studies are particularly prone to biased results. These biases are discussed in the next section.

BIAS IN CASE CONTROL STUDIES

The word "experimental" is generally used by epidemiologists to refer to clinical trials, but there are elements of experimental manipulation in case control studies as well. In case control research, the investigators manipulate the comparison groups, rather than the exposure or treatment, whereas nature determines who becomes a case and who is fortunate enough to remain a noncase or control in a cohort or prevalence study. This element of manipulation is a necessary evil because if the investigator cannot achieve comparability of cases and controls, the findings will be dismissed.

Cases and controls are comparable if they were equally likely to have been exposed to the factor of interest under the assumption that the exposure is unrelated to the disease. In other words, to be comparable, cases and controls must seem to have had an equal chance of being exposed. For example, the opportunity to have received postmenopausal estrogens (discussed earlier) would presumably be greater among women who have received regular medical care and perhaps still greater among women who have received regular gynecologic care; thus, comparability as defined previously would be more acceptable if both cases and controls had similar medical care experiences. But how similar should they be? If one insists that cases and controls have the same doctor, the study may be nullified if that doctor systematically either prescribes or does not prescribe estrogens to all postmenopausal patients.

Therefore, ensuring comparability between cases and controls requires the careful consideration of the circumstances under which an individual becomes exposed.

Selecting Cases

The cases in case control research should if possible be new (incident) cases, not existing (prevalent) ones. The reasons are based on the concepts discussed in Chapter 4, frequency. Disease is prevalent, at a point in time, in relation to both the incidence and duration of that disease. Duration is in turn determined by the rate at which patients leave the disease state (because of recovery or death) or persist in it because of a slow course or successful palliation. It follows from these relationships that risk factors for prevalent disease are risk factors for both incidence and duration; the relative contributions of the two cannot be distinguished. Thus, an exposure that causes a particularly lethal form of the disease, thereby lowering the proportion of prevalent cases that are exposed, would result in a lowered relative risk, suggesting that it protects against developing the disease.

Of course, if one can be sure that the duration of disease is about the same in exposed and nonexposed people, then the odds ratio obtained from a prevalence study might be a fair estimate of relative risk for developing disease.

Selecting Controls

A major potential for bias exists in case control studies because the controls are selected by the investigators. Which controls are appropriate in relation to the cases? The fundamental question is: Are controls as likely to be exposed as cases, for reasons other than having the disease? Any systematic differences between cases and controls that might be related to exposure could distort the odds ratio, making it an inaccurate estimate of the true risk.

There are several strategies for choosing the right controls. First, it is possible to minimize selection bias by selecting both cases and controls from unbiased samples of the same population. If cases are a complete sample of all cases arising in a defined population, then controls can be a random sample of all the other people in the same population. Alternatively, cases and controls can be unbiased samples of the same cohort— that is, a more selected, generally smaller group of people observed over time. This strategy is called a *population-based* or *nested* (in a cohort) *case control study.* Controls should meet the same inclusion/exclusion criteria as the cases and be sampled from the population or cohort at about the same time as the case arose.

Example—Does habitual, vigorous physical activity protect against primary cardiac arrest in people without apparent heart disease? Siscovick et al. conducted a population-based case control study to answer this question (11). Cases were selected from 1250 people living in Seattle and suburban King County, Washington, who had suffered out-of-hospital primary cardiac arrest (PCA) during a defined period of time. Cases were chosen from paramedic reports; paramedics attended nearly all instances of PCA in the area at the time.

Controls were selected by dialing randomly selected telephone numbers in the same area; most people in the area had telephones in their homes.

Both cases and controls had to meet criteria for entry: age 25–75 years, no clinically recognizable heart disease, no prior disease that limited activity, and a spouse who could provide information about habitual exercise—the exposure of interest. Controls were matched to cases on age, sex, marital status, and urban or suburban residence. Spouses of both cases and controls were asked about leisure-time activity. (Most physical exertion in these people took place outside of working hours.)

The results, based on 163 eligible cases and controls, confirmed previous studies. The risk of PCA was 65–75% lower in persons with high-intensity leisure-time activity, compared to more sedentary people (11).

Although selecting cases and controls from a defined population or cohort is ideal, selecting from hospitals is more feasible. But studying people in institutions is also more fallible because hospitalized patients are usually a biased sample of all people in the community, the people to whom the results should apply.

A second set of strategies for having controls who are comparable to cases include the ones presented in the chapter on prognosis: restriction matching, stratification, and adjustment. Matching poses the greatest challenges, and will be discussed here.

Cases can be *matched* with controls so that for each case one or more controls are selected who possess characteristics in common with the case. Researchers commonly match for age, race, and sex because these are frequently related to disease. But matching often extends beyond these demographic characteristics when other factors are known to be important.

If performed properly, matching maximizes the information obtainable from a set of cases and controls because it reduces differences between groups in determinants of disease other than the one being considered and thereby allows for a more powerful (sensitive) test of association. But matching carries a risk. If the investigator happens to match on a factor that is itself related to exposure, there is an increased chance that the matched case and control will have the same history of exposure. For example, if cases and controls were matched for hot flashes, which are commonly treated with estrogens, it would increase the likelihood that the two groups would have similar exposure to estrogens. This process, called *overmatching*, can result in a falsely low estimate of relative risk.

A third strategy is to choose more than one control group.[c] Because of the difficulties attending the selection of truly comparable control groups, a systematic error in the odds ratio may arise for any one of them. A way to guard against this possibility is to choose more than one control group, particularly if they are drawn from different sources. One approach used when cases are drawn from a hospital is to choose one control group from other patients in the same hospital and a second control group from the neighborhoods in which the cases live. If similar odds ratios are obtained using different control groups, this is evidence against bias because it is unlikely that bias would affect otherwise dissimilar groups to the same extent. If the estimates of relative risks are different, that is a signal that one or both are biased, and an opportunity exists to investigate where the bias lies.

Example—In a case control study of estrogen and endometrial cancer, cases were identified from a single teaching hospital. Two control groups were selected: one from among gynecologic admissions to the same hospital and the second from a random sample of women living in the area served by the hospital.

Table 10.3 shows the distribution of various characteristics, including estrogen use, among these three groups. Note that the presence of other diseases, such as hypertension, diabetes, or gallbladder disease, was much more common among the two hospital groups, presumably reflecting the various forces that lead to hospitalization. Despite these differences, the two control groups reported much less long-term estrogen use than did the cases and yielded very similar odds ratios (4.1 and 3.6).

The authors concluded that "this consistency of results with two very different

---

[c] Choosing two or more control groups per case group is different from choosing two or more controls per case. The former is, in a sense, similar to performing two or more studies. Each must stand on its own, although the information from one may help interpret the other. On the other hand, choosing two or more cases per control is done to increase statistical power (or precision of estimate of relative risk) when a fixed and limited number of cases is available, but as is usually the case, there are many potential controls. In general, using two controls per case results in small but useful gains in power (but of course more patients to study). At three controls per case, there is a small additional gain; there is no useful advantage to adding more controls per case beyond three or four.

Table 10.3

Characteristics of Cases and Two Control Groups: A Case Control Study of Estrogen Exposure and Endometrial Cancer[a]

CHARACTERISTIC	CASES	GYNECOLOGY CONTROLS	COMMUNITY CONTROLS
No. of subjects	186	153	236
Mean age	60	60	55
% nulliparous	27	14	16
% obese	52	40	31
% hypertensive	51	48	34
% diabetic	19	17	7
% gallbladder disease	18	26	12
% long-term (3.5 yr) estrogen use	20	3	7

[a] Adapted from Hulka BS, Fowler WC Jr, Kaufman DG, Greenberg BG, Hogue CJR, Berger GS, Pulliam CC: Am J Obstet Gynecol 137:92–101, 1980.

comparison groups suggests that neither is significantly biased and that the results ... are reasonably accurate" (12).

A somewhat different approach is to choose one set of controls to probe for possible biases in another. Thus, if the investigator suspects from what is already known about exposure and disease that using a particular control group might result in an artificially high odds ratio, he or she might select another group of controls that would seem in danger of producing a too low odds ratio. If estimates of risks from the two different control groups are not very different, then the concerns were unfounded.

Options for selecting cases and controls are summarized in Figure 10.4. If cases are all (or a representative sample of all cases) in a defined population, then controls should be too—and so much the better. If cases are a biased sample of all cases, as they are in most hospitals, then controls should be selected with similar biases.

Measuring Exposure

Even if selection bias can be avoided in choosing cases and controls, the investigator faces problems associated with validly measuring exposure after the disease or outcome has occurred—that is, avoiding measurement bias. Three kinds of measurement bias can occur.

1. The presence of the outcome directly affects the exposure.
2. The presence of the outcome affects the subject's recollection of the exposure.
3. The presence of the outcome affects the measurement or recording of the exposure.

We will illustrate these, again using the example of estrogen and endometrial cancer.

First, it has been postulated that because endometrial cancer most

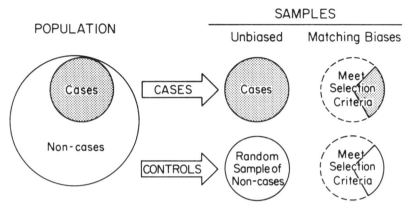

Figure 10.4. Two strategies for selecting cases and controls from the general population: unbiased samples and samples with matching biases.

commonly presents to physicians as postmenopausal vaginal bleeding and estrogens are sometimes prescribed as treatment for postmenopausal bleeding, this therapeutic use of estrogens accounts for their association with endometrial cancer. Although this sequence of events has proven to be uncommon, it represents one way in which the presence of an outcome can lead to exposure, rather than vice versa.

Second, people with a disease may recall exposure differently from those without the disease. With all the publicity surrounding the possible risks of estrogen use, it is entirely possible that victims of endometrial cancer would remember their previous drug histories more accurately than non-victims or even overestimate their estrogen use. The influence of disease on memory status, called recall bias, is illustrated by a study of the possible familial aggregation of rheumatoid arthritis (13). As shown in Table 10.4, patients with rheumatoid arthritis were more likely to give a family history of rheumatoid arthritis than were controls. However, this association was not present when family histories given by the unaffected siblings of the rheumatoid arthritis cases were compared with those of controls. As we are all well aware, it is natural for sick people to seek explanations for their misfortunes; and backward research, as in case control or prevalence studies provides an opportunity for doing so.

Critical readers should look for two protections against biased remembering. First, there should be alternative sources of the same information, whether written documents, such as medical or other records, or interviews with relatives or other knowledgable individuals. Second, the specific purpose of the study should be concealed from the study subjects. It would be unethical not to inform subjects of the general nature of the study question. But to provide detailed information to subjects about the specific hypotheses could so bias the resulting information obtained as to commit another breach of ethics—involving subjects in a worthless research project.

Table 10.4

Effect of Outcome on Measurement of Exposure: Reported Family History of Rheumatoid Arthritis according to whether or not the Reporter has the Disease[a]

FAMILY HISTORY OF ARTHRITIS	CONTROLS	RHEUMATOID ARTHRITIS (RA) PATIENTS	SIBLINGS OF RA PATIENTS
	%	%	%
Neither parent	55	27	50
One parent	37	58	42
Both parents	8	15	8

[a] Adapted from Sackett DL: *J Chron Dis* 32:51–63, 1979; and Schull WJ, Cobb S: *J Chron Dis* 22:217–222, 1969.

The third problem, whether the presence of the outcome influences the way in which the exposure is measured or recorded, should be understandable to all students of physical diagnosis. If a gynecology resident admitting a woman with endometrial cancer to the hospital is aware of a possible link between estrogen use and endometrial cancer one could expect the resident to question the patient more intensely about previous hormone use and to record the information more carefully. Interviewers who are aware of a possible relationship between exposure and disease and also the outcome status of the interviewee would be remarkable indeed if they conducted identical interviews for cases and controls. The protections against these sources of bias are the same as those mentioned above: multiple sources of information and blinding the data gatherers, i.e., keeping them in the dark as to the hypothesis under study.

Scientific Standards for Case Control Research

It has been suggested that one should judge the validity of a case control study by first considering how a randomized controlled trial of the same question would have been conducted (14). Of course, one could not actually do the study that way. But a randomized controlled trial would be the scientific standard against which to consider the effects of the various compromises that are inherent in a case control study.

Thus, if one would enter into a trial only those patients who could take the experimental intervention if it were offered, so in a case control study one would select cases and controls who could have been exposed. For example, a study of whether exogenous estrogens are a cause of endometrial cancer would include women who had seen physicians (and so could have received a prescription) and had no contraindications to taking exogenous estrogens. Similarly, both cases and controls should have been subjected to equal efforts to discover endometrial cancer if it were present. These and other parallels between clinical trials and case control studies can be exploited when trying to think through just what could go wrong, how serious a problem is it, and what can be done about it.

There have also been efforts to set out criteria for sound case control studies (15). To apply these guidelines requires an indepth understanding of the many possible determinants of exposure and disease, as well as the detection of both, in actual clinical situations.

SUMMARY

Rare diseases, because they occur so infrequently, must often be studied using less than optimal research designs. Case reports are studies of just a few patients, e.g., ≤10. They have been a useful means of surveillance for rare disease, describing rare presentations of disease, and understanding the mechanisms of disease. However, case reports are of little help in characterizing the frequency of disease, and they are particularly prone to bias and chance. Case series describe patients at a single point in time. They suffer from the absence of a reference group with which to compare the experience of the cases.

In case control studies, a group of cases is compared with a similar group of noncases (controls). This approach has seen increasing use in the study of rare disease. Its advantage resides in the ability to assemble cases from treatment centers as opposed to finding them or waiting for them to develop in a defined population at risk. Thus, case control studies are much less expensive and much quicker to perform than cohort studies. It is not possible to compute incidences from case control studies nor can relative risk be obtained directly. However, relative risk can be estimated by the odds ratio. The disadvantages of the case control design all relate to its considerable susceptibility to bias. This problem is most related to two characteristics of case control research. First, the groups to be compared are selected by the researcher and are not constituted naturally; second, the exposure is measured after the disease has already occurred.

Given the vulnerability of case control studies to bias, what place do they have in clinical epidemiologic research? To some, case control studies are unscientific, illogical, and a curse. To others, they are viewed as the essential first step in studying most medically important questions. There is nearly universal agreement that cohort studies provide stronger, more valid evidence and, if feasible, are the design of choice. But with appropriate attention to possible sources of bias, case control studies can provide a valid and efficient method to answer many clinical questions, particularly those involving rare diseases.

REFERENCES

1. National Center for Health Statistics: *Prevalence of Selected Chronic Respiratory Conditions: United States 1970.* (Series 10, No. 84) U.S. Department of Health, Education, and Welfare, Rockville, MD.
2. Lelah T, Harris L, Avery C, Brook R: Asthma in children and adults: assessing the quality of medical care using short-term outcome measures. In Avery A, Lelah T, Solomon N, Harris L, Brook R, Greenfield S, Ware J Jr, Avery C (eds): *Quality of Medical Care Assessment Using Outcome Measures: Eight Disease-Specific Applications.* Santa Monica, CA, Rand Corp., 1976.

3. Fletcher RH, Fletcher SW: Clinical research in general medicine journals: A 30-year perspective. *N Engl J Med* 301:180–183, 1979.
4. Klatskin G, Kimberg DV: Recurrent hepatitis attributable to halothane sensitization in an anesthetist. *N Engl J Med* 280:515–522, 1969.
5. Dietz PE: Sampling bias in the case report: The example of post mortem Cesarean section. Presented at Robert Wood Johnson Clinical Scholars Program National Meeting, 1979.
6. Mulvihill JJ: Clinical ecogenetics. Cancer in families. *N Engl J Med* 312:1569–1570, 1985.
7. Berkson J: Limitations of the application of fourfold table analysis to hospital data. *Biomed Bull* 2:47–53, 1946.
8. Jaffe HW, Bregman DJ, Selik RM: Acquired immune deficiency syndrome in the United States: The first 1,000 cases. *J Infectious Dis* 148:339–345, 1983.
9. Feinstein AR: The bias caused by high values of incidence for p_1 in the odds ratio assumption that $1 - P_1 \simeq 1$. *J Chron Dis* 39:485–487, 1986.
10. Cole P: The evolving case control study. *J Chron Dis* 32:15–27, 1979.
11. Siscovick DS, Weiss NS, Hallstrom AP, Inui TS, Peterson DR: Physical activity and primary cardiac arrest. *JAMA* 248:3113–3117, 1982.
12. Hulka BS, Fowler WC Jr, Kaufman DG, Greenberg BG, Hogue CJR, Berger GS, Pulliam CC: Estrogen and endometrial cancer: Cases and two control groups from North Carolina. *Am J Obstet Gynecol* 137:92–101, 1980.
13. Sackett DL: Bias in analytic research. *J Chron Dis* 32:51–63, 1979.
14. Feinstein AR, Horwitz RI: Double standards, scientific methods and epidemiologic research. *N Engl J Med* 307:1611–1617, 1982.
15. Horwitz R, Feinstein AR: Methodologic standards and contradictory results in case-control research. *Am J Med* 66:556–564, 1979.

SUGGESTED READINGS

Feinstein AR: Clinical biostatistics XX: The epidemiologic trohoc, the ablative risk ratio, and 'retrospective research.' *Clin Pharmacol Ther* 14:291–307, 1973.
Feinstein AR, Horwitz RI, Spitzer WO, Battista RN: Coffee and pancreatic cancer: the problems of etiologic science and epidemiological case-control research. *JAMA* 246:957–961, 1981.
Feinstein AR, Horwitz RI: Double standards, scientific methods, and epidemiologic research. *N Engl J Med* 307:1611–1617, 1982.
Hayden GF, Kramer MS, Horwitz RI: The case-control study. A practical review for the clinician. *JAMA* 247:326–331, 1982.
Horwitz RI, Feinstein AR: Methodologic standards and contradictory results in case-control research. *Am J Med* 66:556–564, 1979.
Ibrahim MA, Spitzer WO: *The Case-Control Study: Consensus and Controversy.* New York, Pergamon Press, 1979 (also published in a special issue of *J Chronic Dis* 32:1–144, 1979).
Rothman KJ: *Modern Epidemiology.* Boston, Little, Brown and Co, 1986.
Schlesselman JJ: *Case-Control Studies. Design, Conduct, Analysis.* New York, Oxford University Press, 1982.

APPENDIX 10.1. MAIN QUESTIONS FOR DETERMINING THE VALIDITY OF STUDIES OF RISK FACTORS (OR CAUSES) USING A CASE CONTROL APPROACH[a]

1. Were cases:
   a. Entered in the study *at onset of disease?*

---

[a] The questions are not meant to be all-inclusive nor to replace independent, critical thinking. They are rough guidelines, including only the most basic elements of a sound study.

(If prevalent cases, consider how differences in duration of disease, if related to exposure, could affect estimate of relative risk)
   b. *Described concerning criteria for diagnosis?*
2. *Were controls comparable to cases* as likely to be exposed for reasons other than being a case?
   One or more of the following strategies can be used:
   a. Select sample of cases and controls from the same, defined population.
   b. If cases are biased sample of all cases in the population, select controls with similar biases (opportunity for exposure), i.e., similar setting, inclusion/exclusion criteria, time of entry, etc.
   c. Control for the effects of known extraneous variables by restriction, matching, stratified analysis, and/or mathematical adjustment.
   d. Compare results from more than one control group, selected to uncover potential bias.
3. Have cases and controls undergone *similar efforts to detect the disease* (particularly if the disease can have a long "silent," subclinical phase)?
4. *Was exposure*:
   a. *Defined*: type dose, duration, etc.?
   b. *Know to precede disease?*
   c. *Recorded without bias* related to disease status?

chapter 11

CAUSE

Some years ago, our medical students were presented a study of the relationship between the cigarette smoking habits of obstetricians and the vigor of babies they delivered. Infant vigor was measured by an Apgar score; a high score (9–10) indicated that the baby was healthy, whereas a lower score indicated the baby might be in trouble and require close monitoring. The study suggested that smoking by obstetricians (not in the delivery suite!) had an adverse effect on Apgar scores in newborns.

The medical students were then asked to comment on what was wrong with this study, with its unexpected results indicating that obstetricians' smoking caused unhealthy infants. After many suggestions, someone finally said that the conclusion simply did not make sense.

It was then acknowledged that, although the study was real, the "exposure" and "disease" had been altered for the presentation. Instead of comparing smoking habits of obstetricians with Apgar scores of newborns, the study was published in 1843 by Oliver Wendell Holmes (then Professor of Anatomy and Physiology, and later Dean of Harvard Medical School) and concerned hand washing habits by obstetricians and subsequent puerperal sepsis in mothers. His observations led him to conclude: "The disease known as puerperal fever is so far contagious, as to be frequently carried from patient to patient by physicians and nurses" (1).

One mid-19th century response to Holmes' assertion that unwashed hands caused puerperal fever was remarkably similar to that of the medical students: The findings made no sense. "I prefer to attribute them (puerperal sepsis cases) to accident, or Providence, of which I can form a conception, rather than to contagion of which I cannot form any clear idea, at least as to this particular malady" (1). This response was written by the prestigious Dr. Charles D. Meigs, Professor of Midwifery and the Diseases of Women and Children at Jefferson Medical College.[a]

---

[a] This example thanks to Dr. John Hoey, Faculty of Medicine, McGill University, Montreal.

Holmes and Meigs were confronted with a question of cause and effect. Holmes was convinced by his data that the spread of puerperal sepsis was caused by obstetricians not washing their hands between deliveries. He could not, however, supply the pathogenetic mechanism by which hand washing was related to the disease. Meigs, therefore, remained unconvinced that the cause of puerperal sepsis had been established (and presumably did not bother to wash his hands).

Clinicians frequently are confronted with information about possible cause-and-effect relationships. In fact, most of this book has been about methods used to establish causation, although we have not called special attention to the term.

In this chapter, we will review concepts of cause in clinical medicine. We will then outline the kinds of evidence that, when present, strengthen the likelihood that an association represents a cause-and-effect relationship. Finally, we will deal briefly with a kind of research design not yet considered in this book: studies in which exposure to a possible cause is known only for groups and not specifically for individuals in the groups.

CONCEPTS OF CAUSE

Websters' Dictionary defines *cause* as "something that brings about an effect or a result" (2). In medical textbooks, cause is usually discussed under such headings as "etiology," "pathogenesis," or "mechanisms."

Cause is primarily important to practicing physicians in guiding their approach to three clinical tasks: prevention, diagnosis, and treatment. The clinical example at the beginning of this chapter illustrates how knowledge of cause-and-effect relationships can lead to successful preventive strategies. Likewise, when we periodically check patients' blood pressures, we are reacting to arguments that hypertension causes morbidity and mortality and that treatment of hypertension causes a reduction in these events. The diagnostic process, especially in infectious disease, frequently involves a search for the causative agent. Less directly, this process often depends on information about cause when the presence of risk factors is used to identify groups of patients in whom disease prevalence is high (Chapter 3). Finally, the knowledge of (or at least hope for) a cause-and-effect relationship underlies every therapeutic maneuver in clinical medicine. Why give penicillin unless we think it will cause a cure of pneumococcal pneumonia? Or why advise a patient with metastatic cancer to undergo chemotherapy unless we believe the antimetabolite will cause a regression of metastases and a prolongation of survival, comfort, and/or ability to carry on daily activities.

By and large, clinicians are more interested in treatable or reversible than immutable causes. Researchers, on the other hand, might also be interested in studying causal factors for which no efficacious treatment or prevention exists in hopes of developing methods of prevention and treatments in the future.

Single and Multiple Causes

In 1882, 40 years after the Holmes-Meigs confrontation, Koch set forth his postulates for determining that an infectious agent is the cause of a disease:

1. The organism must be present in every case of the disease.
2. The organism must be isolated and grown in pure culture.
3. The organism must, when inoculated into a susceptible animal, cause the specific disease.
4. The organism must then be recovered from the animal and identified.

Koch's postulates contributed greatly to the concept of cause in medicine. Before Koch, it was believed that many different bacteria caused any given disease. The application of his postulates helped bring order out of chaos and enabled important scientific advances to be made. They are still useful today. For example, Koch's postulates were the basis for the discovery in 1977 that Legionnaire's disease is caused by a gram negative bacterium.

For many diseases, however, cause cannot be established by means of Koch's postulates. Basic to his approach was the assumption that a particular disease had one cause, and a particular cause results in one disease. Would that all diseases were so simple! Smoking causes lung cancer, chronic obstructive pulmonary disease, peptic ulcers, bladder cancer, and coronary artery disease. On the other hand, coronary artery disease has multiple causes, including cigarette smoking, hypertension, and hypercholesterolemia. It is also possible to have coronary artery disease without any of these known risk factors being present.

Usually many factors act together to cause disease. This process has been called the "web of causation" (3). Koch's postulates are useful only in those special circumstances in which one particular cause dominates (perhaps because the other determinants of disease are already present, but insufficient in themselves to cause disease) and when that cause is physically transmissible.

Proximity of Cause to Effect

When biomedical scientists study causes of disease, they usually search for the underlying pathogenetic mechanism or final common pathway of disease. It is our impression that most clinicians accept this as the fundamental approach to determining cause-and-effect relationships. Certainly basic biomedical research aimed at elucidating pathogenetic causes of disease has played a crucial part in the advancement of medical science in this century. However, the occurrence of disease is also determined by less specific, more remote causes, such as genetic, environmental, or behavioral factors, that occur earlier in the chain of events leading to a disease. These are sometimes referred to as "origins" of disease and are more likely to be investigated by epidemiologists. These less specific and more remote causes of disease are the risk factors discussed in Chapter 5.

Unfortunately, if the pathogenetic mechanism is not clear, it is sometimes assumed that the cause of a disease is not known. Yet, knowledge of risk factors may lead to very effective treatments and preventions that can be applied without knowing the pathogenetic mechanism of a disease. (Thus, Holmes was right in his assertion that obstetricians should wash their hands, even though he had little notion of bacteria.) To view cause in medicine exclusively as cellular and subcellular processes restricts the possibilities for useful clinical interventions.

The following is an example of a disease with a rich array of causes, most of which are amenable to interventions that either prevent or reverse the disease.

Example—Koch's postulates were originally used to establish that tuberculosis is caused by innoculation of the acid-fast bacillus, *mycobacterium tuberculosis*, into susceptible hosts. The final common pathway of tuberculosis is the invasion of host tissue by the bacteria. From a pathogenetic perspective, conquering the disease required antibiotics or vaccines that were effective against the organism. Through biomedical research efforts, both have been developed.

However, the development of the disease tuberculosis is far more complex. Other important causes are the susceptibility of the host and the degree of exposure (Fig. 11.1). In fact, these causes determine whether invasion of host tissue can occur.

Some clinicians would be hesitant to label host susceptibility and level of exposure as causes of tuberculosis, but they are very important components of cause. In fact, social and economic factors influencing host susceptibility may have played a more prominent role in the decline in tuberculosis rates in developed countries than treatments developed through the biomedical-pathogenetic research model. Figure 11.2 shows that the death rate from tuberculosis had dropped dramatically long before antibiotics were introduced. (The vaccine came even later.)

Another example of the importance of both pathogenetic and epidemiologic approaches to cause is the recent decline in deaths from coronary artery disease in the United States. Over the past decade, the death rate

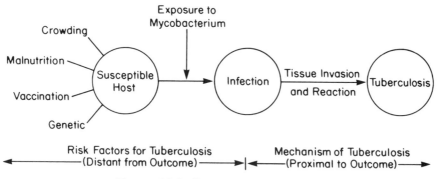

Figure 11.1. Causes of tuberculosis.

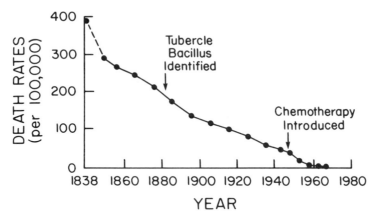

Figure 11.2. Declining death rate from respiratory tuberculosis. (Redrawn from McKeown T: *The Role of Medicine: Dream, Mirage or Nemesis.* London, Nuffield Provincial Hospital Trust, 1976.

from coronary artery disease has dropped over 30%. This decline accompanied decreased exposure, in the population as a whole, to several risk factors for cardiovascular disease: A larger proportion of people with hypertension are being treated effectively, middle-aged men are smoking less, and cholesterol consumption has declined. These developments were, at least in part, the result of both epidemiologic and biomedical studies and have spared tens of thousands of lives per year. It is doubtful that they would have occurred without the understanding of both the proximal mechanisms and the more remote origins of cardiovascular disease.

Interaction of Multiple Causes

When more than one cause act together, their effects are not necessarily simply additive. Often, the resulting risk is greater than would be expected by simply adding the effects of the separate causes.

Example—Figure 11.3 shows the probability of developing cardiovascular disease over an 8-year period among men aged 40. Those men who did not smoke cigarettes, had low serum cholesterol values, and had low systolic blood pressure readings were at low risk of developing disease (12/1000). Risk increased, in the range of 20 to 61/1000, when the various factors were present individually. But when all three factors were present, the risk of cardiovascular disease (317/1000) was almost three times greater than the sum of the individual risks (4).

Elucidation of cause is more difficult when many factors play a part than when a single one predominates. However, when multiple causative factors are present and interact, it may be possible to make a substantial impact on a patient's health by changing only one, or a small number, of the causes. Thus, in the previous example, getting patients to give up smoking and treating hypertension might substantially lower the risk of

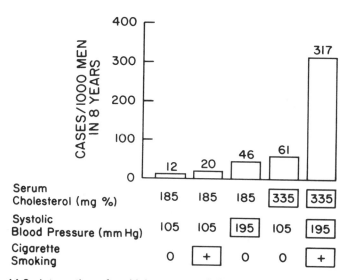

Figure 11.3. Interaction of multiple causes of disease: risk of developing cardio-vascular disease in men according to the level of several risk factors alone and in combination—abnormal values enclosed in boxes. (Redrawn from Kannel WB: Preventive cardiology. *Postgrad Med* 61:74–85, 1977.)

Table 11.1

Estimated Relative Risk of Myocardial Infarction from Oral Contraceptive Use according to Cigarette Smoking[a]

CIGARETTE SMOKING	ORAL CONTRACEPTIVE USE	
	NO	YES
None	1.0	4.5
1–24/day	3.4	3.7
>25/day	7.0	39.0

[a] From Shapiro S, Slone D, Rosenberg L, Kaufman DW, Stolley PD, Miettinen OS: Oral-contraceptive use in relation to myocardial infarction. *Lancet* 1: 743–747, 1979.

developing cardiovascular disease in men, even in the continuing presence of other causative factors.

Effect modification is present when the strength of the cause-and-effect relationship between two variables is different according to the level of some third variable, called an *effect modifier.*[b]

Example—Does cigarette smoking modify the relationship between oral contraceptive use and myocardial infarction? Shapiro et al. addressed this question with a case control study. They recorded oral contraceptive use and cigarette smoking in 234 premenopausal women with a first myocardial infarction and 1742 hospital controls (5). The results are shown in Table 11.1.

---

[b] Effect modification can be thought of in terms of either relative or attributable risk. The mathematical expression for it is "statistical interaction."

Although oral contraceptive use was associated with an increased risk, the risk of myocardial infarction was particularly high among oral contraceptive users who smoked—that is, smoking modified the relationship between oral contraceptive use and myocardial infarction.

ESTABLISHING CAUSE: STUDIES OF INDIVIDUALS

In clinical medicine, it is not possible to prove causal relationships beyond any doubt. It is only possible to increase one's conviction of a cause-and-effect relationship, by means of empiric evidence, to the point where, for all intents and purposes, cause is established. Conversely, evidence against a cause can be mounted until a cause-and-effect relationship becomes implausible.

These principles are true even for clinical applications of well-established laboratory findings. Although more certainty can be attached to observations made in the laboratory under highly controlled conditions, a biologic mechanism established in the laboratory cannot be assumed to apply to intact patients. The particular mechanism that is characterized under carefully controlled conditions may be overpowered by other, competing mechanisms that are not yet understood.

Cause-and-effect relationships for humans, therefore, must ultimately be established in intact humans. In order to do so, the possibility of a postulated cause-and-effect relationship should be examined in as many different ways as possible.

Association and Cause

Two factors—the suspected cause and the effect—obviously must appear to be associated if they are to be considered cause and effect. However, not all associations are causal. Figure 11.4 outlines other kinds of associa-

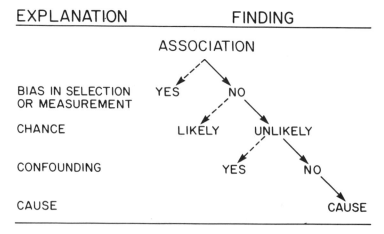

Figure 11.4. Association and cause.

tions that must be excluded. First, a decision must be made as to whether an apparent association between a purported cause and an effect is real or merely an artifact because of bias or random variation. Selection and measurement biases and the role of chance are most likely to give rise to apparent associations that in reality do not exist. If these problems can be considered unlikely, a true association exists. But before deciding that the association is causal, it is necessary to know if the association occurs indirectly, through another (confounding) factor, or directly. If confounding is not found, a causal relationship is likely. However, one should always keep in mind that at some future time another factor may be found that is more directly causal. For example, when it was found that jaundice followed injection of neoarsphenamine for syphilis, the drug was considered responsible. Later, the jaundice was found to be secondary to hepatitis resulting from the use of unclean syringes to inject neoarsphenamine, not the drug itself. Thus, factors that are considered causes at one time are sometimes found to be indirectly related to disease later, when more evidence is available.

Hierarchy of Research Designs

The most important evidence for a cause-and-effect relationship is the strength of the research design used to establish the relationship.

Well-conducted randomized controlled trials, with adequate numbers of patients; blinding of therapists, patients, and researchers; and carefully standardized methods of measurement and analysis are the best evidence for a cause-and-effect relationship. As pointed out in Chapter 7, the reason why randomized controlled trials are the most powerful way of establishing cause-and-effect relationships in clinical investigations is that they are best suited to study the unique effects of a single factor. They guard against differences in the groups being compared, both for factors already known to be important, which can be overcome by means other than a randomized controlled trial, and for unknown confounding factors.

We ordinarily use randomized controlled trials to provide evidence about cause-and-effect relationships for treatments and prevention. At least theoretically, such trials could also be used to show that a particular agent causes a disease. However, practically speaking, it is usually not possible to use them for this purpose. Although potentially helpful agents may be assigned at random, at least to some patients, most potentially harmful agents or risk factors cannot. To do so would be unethical, because patients who enter these trials could only do worse than they would have done without the trial. Moreover, even the removal of potential risk factors is rarely possible. For example, although one can randomize laboratory animals to smoking and nonsmoking groups, it is certainly not possible to do so with humans. Then too, there are problems of long latent periods and large numbers of subjects needed to answer most questions about cause-and-effect relationships in clinical medicine. Because of all these problems, randomized controlled trials are rarely feasible when studying causes of disease. Observational studies must be used instead.

In general, the further one must depart from randomized trials, the less the research design protects against possible biases and the weaker the evidence is for a cause-and-effect relationship. Well-conducted cohort studies are the next best design to experiments, because they can be conducted to minimize the effects of selection and measurement biases, as well as known confounding biases. Cross-sectional studies are vulnerable because they provide no direct evidence of the sequence of events. True prevalence surveys, cross-sectional studies of a defined population, guard against selection bias, but are subject to measurement and confounding biases. As pointed out in Chapter 10, case control studies are vulnerable to selection bias as well. Weakest of all are cases series because they have no defined population and no comparison group.

Of course, this hierarchy of research designs is only a rough guide, based on extent of susceptibility to bias. The manner in which an individual study is performed can do a great deal to increase or decrease its validity, regardless of the type of design used.

Summarizing the Evidence for or against Cause

When experiments are not possible and only observational studies are available, deciding whether something is a cause requires judgment, based on all the evidence. In 1965, the British statistician, Sir Austin Bradford-Hill, proposed a set of criteria that could be used to guide decisions about whether an environmental factor is a cause of disease (Table 11.2) (6). By

Table 11.2
Evidence that an Association is Cause and Effect[a]

CRITERION	COMMENTS
Temporality	Cause precedes effect
Strength	Large relative risk
Dose-response	Larger exposures to cause associated with higher rates of disease
Reversibility	Reduction in exposure associated with lower rates of disease
Consistency	Repeatedly observed by different persons, in different places, circumstances, and times
Biologic plausibility	Makes sense, according to biologic knowledge of the time
Specificity	One cause leads to one effect
Analogy	Cause-and-effect relationship already established for a similar exposure/disease

[a] Modified from Hill AB: The environment and disease. Association and causation. *Proc Roy Soc Med* 58: 295–300, 1965.

examining the pattern of information, evidence for causality can be strengthened or eroded. This way of summarizing the evidence for causality has been widely used, sometimes with modifications, ever since. We will comment briefly on the individual criteria. They are not all of equal weight.

1. **Temporal relationships between cause and effect**
   Causes should obviously precede effects. This fundamental principle seems self-evident, but it can be overlooked when interpreting cross-sectional studies and some case control studies, in which both purported causes and effects are measured at the same point in time. In these two types of studies, it is often assumed that one variable precedes another without actually establishing that this is so. The controversy about whether estrogen therapy causes endometrial cancer is an example of this problem, as pointed out in Chapter 10. Some investigators argue that the assumption in case control studies that estrogen therapy leads to endometrial cancer, which then is discovered because of postmeno-pausal uterine bleeding, may be in error. They argue that, because exogenous estrogens are used to treat postmenopausal bleeding, it is possible that endometrial cancer causes uterine bleeding, which then leads to estrogen therapy being prescribed. If the endometrial cancer is diagnosed after estrogen therapy is begun, it would then seem that estrogens preceded the cancer, but such a conclusion would be incorrect. (Subsequent studies have shown that the latter possibility could not explain all of the observed odds ratio, but the example does illustrate that temporal sequence may not be clear in noncohort studies of cause-and-effect relationships.)
   Although it is absolutely necessary for a cause to precede an effect temporal sequence alone is weak evidence for cause.

2. **Strength of the association**
   A strong association between a purported cause and an effect, as expressed by a large relative risk or odds ratio, is better evidence for a causal relationship than a weak association. Thus, the 4- to 16-fold increase of lung cancer among smokers, compared to nonsmokers, in many different prospective studies is much stronger evidence that smoking causes lung cancer than the findings in these same studies that smoking may be related to renal cancer, where the relative risks are much smaller (1.1–1.6) (7). Similarly, that the relative risk of hepatitis B infection for hepatocellular cancer is nearly 300 leaves little doubt that the virus is a cause of liver cancer (8). Bias can sometimes result in large relative risks. However, unrecognized bias is less likely to produce large relative risks than small ones.

3. **Dose-response relationships**
   A dose-response relationship is present when varying amounts of the purported cause are related to varying amounts of the effect. If a dose-response relationship can be demonstrated, it strengthens the argument for cause and effect. Figure 11.5 shows a clear dose-response curve when lung cancer death rates (responses) are plotted against number of cigarettes smoked (doses).

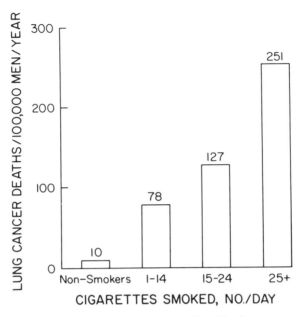

Figure 11.5. Example of a dose-response relationship: lung cancer deaths according to dose of cigarettes in male physicians. (Drawn from Doll R, Peto R: Mortality in relation to smoking: 20 years' observations on male British doctors. *Br Med J* 2:1525–1536, 1976.)

Although a dose-response curve is good evidence for a causal relationship, especially when coupled with a large relative risk, the existence of a dose-response relationship between exposure and disease does not exclude confounding factors. For instance, both the strong association between smoking and lung cancer and the dose-response relationship have been dismissed by the tobacco industry as examples of confounding. According to this argument, there is some unknown variable that both causes people to smoke and increases their risk of developing lung cancer. The more the factor is present, the more both smoking and lung cancer are found—hence, the dose-response relationship. Such an argument is a theoretically plausible explanation for the association between smoking and lung cancer. Short of a randomized controlled trial (which would, on the average, allocate the people with the confounding variable equally to smoking and nonsmoking groups) it is a difficult argument to refute.

4. **Reversible associations**

   A factor is more likely to be a cause of disease if its removal results in a decreased risk of disease, i.e., the association between suspected cause and effect is reversible. For example, people who give up smoking decrease their likelihood of getting lung cancer (Figure 11.6). Nevertheless, confounding can still explain a reversible association. For example, it is still possible (but unlikely) that people willing to give up smoking

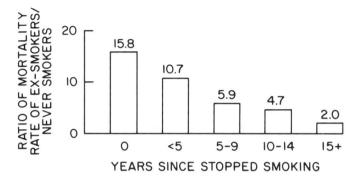

Figure 11.6. Reversible association: declining mortality from lung cancer in ex-cigarette smokers; excludes people who stopped smoking after getting cancer. (Drawn from Doll R, Petro R: Mortality in relation to smoking: 20 years' observations on male British doctors. *Br Med J* 2:1525–1536, 1976.)

have smaller amounts of the unidentified variable than those who continue to smoke.

5. **Consistency**

When several studies, conducted at different times in different settings and with different kinds of patients, all come to the same conclusion, evidence for a causal relationship is strengthened. However, several studies may all make the same mistake. So causation is particularly supported when studies using several different research designs all lead to the same result.

It is often the case that different studies produce different results. Lack of consistency does not necessarily mean that the results of a particular study are invalid. One good study should outweigh several poor ones. We will discuss this concept in the next chapter.

6. **Biologic plausibility**

The biologic plausibility of a purported cause-and-effect relationship (Meigs' criterion, described above) is often given considerable weight when assessing causation. Biologic plausibilty rests on whether the assertion of cause and effect is consistent with our knowledge of the mechanisms of disease as they are currently understood. When we have absolutely no idea how an association might have arisen, we tend to be skeptical that the association is real. Such skepticism often serves us well. For example, the substance Laetrile has been touted as a cure for cancer. However, the scientific community was not convinced that Laetrile would have a beneficial effect on cancer patients. They could think of no biologic reason why it should because the substance is an extract of apricot pits and not chemically related to compounds with known anticancer activity. To "nail down" the issue, Laetrile was finally submitted to a randomized controlled trial in which it was shown that the substance was, in fact, without activity against the cancers studied (9).

It is important to remember, however, that what is considered biologically plausible depends on the state of medical knowledge at the time. In Meig's day, contagious diseases were biologically implausible. Today, a biologically plausible mechanism for puerperal sepsis, the effects of streptococcal infection, has made it easier for us to accept Holmes' observations. On the other hand, the mechanism by which acupuncture causes anesthesia is far less clear. To many, the suggestion that anesthesia is caused by sticking needles into the body and twirling them seems biologically implausible, and so they do not believe in the effectiveness of acupuncture.

In sum, biologic plausibility, when present, strengthens the case for causation. When it is absent, other evidence for causation should be sought. If the other evidence is strong, the lack of biologic plausibility may indicate the limitations of medical knowledge, rather than the lack of a causal association.

7. **Specificity**

Specificity—one cause, one effect—is more often found for acute infectious diseases (such as poliomyelitis and tetanus) and for inborn errors of metabolism (gout, ochronosis, familial hypercholesterolemia, etc). As we pointed out, for chronic, degenerative diseases there are often many causes for the same effect or many effects from the same cause. For example, lung cancer is caused by cigarette smoking, asbestos, and radiation. Cigarettes cause not only lung cancer but also bronchitis, peptic ulcer disease, periodontal disease, and wrinkled skin. So the absence of specificity is not much of a strike against a cause-and-effect relationship.

8. **Analogy**

The cause-and-effect relationship is strengthened if there are examples of well-established causes that are analogous to the one in question. Thus, if we know that a slow virus can cause a chronic, degenerative central nervous system disease (subacute sclerosing panencephalitis) it is easier to accept that another virus might cause degeneration of the immunologic system (acquired immunodeficiency syndrome). In general, however, analogy is weak evidence for cause.

ESTABLISHING CAUSE: STUDIES OF POPULATIONS

Up until now, we have discussed evidence for cause when exposure and disease status are known for each individual in the study. In a different kind of research, most often used for epidemiologic studies of large populations, exposure is known only for the groups, not for the individuals in the groups.

Studies in which exposure to a risk factor is characterized by the average exposure of the group to which individuals belong are called *aggregate risk studies*. Another term is *ecological studies*, because people are classified by the general level of exposure in their environment.

Example—What factors are associated with cardiac mortality in developed countries? St. Leger et al. gathered data on rates of ischemic heart disease mortality in 18 developed countries to explore the contribution of various economic, health services, and dietary variables. One finding that was not anticipated was a strong negative association between ischemic heart disease death and wiñe consumption (Fig. 11.7).

This study raises the hypothesis that alcohol protects against ischemic heart disease. Since then, studies on individuals have shown that levels of serum high density lipoprotein, a protective factor for cardiovascular disease, are increased by alcohol consumption (10).

Aggregate risk studies are rarely definitive in themselves. The main problem is a potential bias called the *ecological fallacy*: As Michael et al. put it, "The ecological fallacy is a foxy, two-faced beast which lurks in the darkened corners of large population studies and tricks unwary readers into accepting unwarranted conclusions" (11). People in a generally exposed group may not themselves be exposed to the risk. Also, exposure may not be the only characteristic that distinguishes people in the exposed group from those in the nonexposed group—that is, there may be confounding factors. Thus, aggregate risk studies are most useful in raising hypotheses, which must then be tested with more rigorous research.

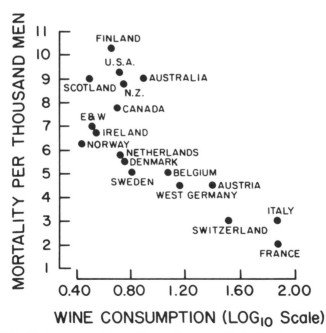

Figure 11.7. Factors associated with cardiac mortality in developed countries with particular reference to the consumption of wine. (St. Leger AS, Cochrane AL, Moore F: Factors associated with cardiac mortality in developed countries with particular reference to the consumption of wine. *Lancet* 1:1017–1020, 1979.)

Time Series Studies

Evidence from aggregate risk studies that a factor is actually responsible for an effect can be strengthened if observations are made at more than two points in time (before and after) and in more than one place. In a *time series study*, the effect is measured at various points in time before and after the purported cause has been introduced. It is then possible to see if the effect varies in a similar fashion. If changes in the purported cause are followed by changes in the purported effect, the association is less likely to be spurious, especially if the association between cause and effect is maintained both while the cause is increasing and decreasing.

Example—In the late 1970s, cases of new and lethal disease, called toxic shock syndrome, began to appear. Patients were usually young women who suffered from acute fever, rash with desquamation, hypotension, mucous membrane inflammation, and clinical or laboratory evidence of abnormalities affecting many systems. The disease often appeared during menstruation.

The frequency of toxic shock syndrome, from 1977 through 1980 is illustrated in Figure 11.8. The tampon suspected of causing toxic shock syndrome was introduced into the market in August 1978 and removed from the market in September 1980. The frequency of reported cases of toxic shock syndrome in the United States varied according to the introduction and withdrawal of the product (12).

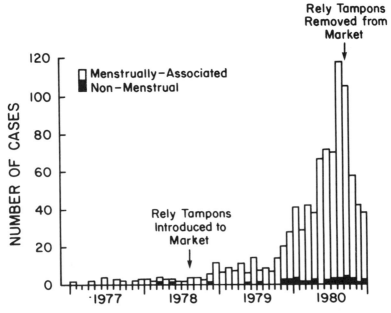

Figure 11.8. Reported cases of toxic shock syndrome in the United States, January 1977 through December 1980, in relation to marketing of *Rely* tampons. (Redrawn from *Morbidity and Mortality* 30:25–28, 1981.)

Although this time series study is stronger evidence for cause than a simple cross-sectional aggregate risk study, it is still possible that women who got toxic shock syndrome may have been those who were not using tampons (ecological fallacy) or they may have been at increasing and then decreasing risk for the syndrome because of other reasons (confounding). These objections were plausible at first; but as it happens in this case, they were ruled out by subsequent studies.

In a *multiple time series study*, the suspected cause has been introduced into several different groups at various times. Measurements of effect are then made among the groups to determine if the effect occurs in the same sequential manner in which the suspected cause was introduced. If the effect regularly follows introduction of the suspected cause at various times and places, there is stronger evidence for cause than if this phenomenon were observed only once because it is even more improbable that the same extraneous factor(s) occurred at the same time in relation to the cause in many different places and eras.

Example—Because there were no randomized controlled trials of cervical cancer screening programs before they became widely accepted, their effectiveness must be evaluated by means of observational studies. A multiple time series study has provided some of the most convincing evidence of their effectiveness. Data were gathered on screening programs begun in the various Canadian provinces at various times during a 10-year period in the 1960s and 1970s. Reductions in mortality regularly followed the introduction of screening programs regardless of time and location. With these data, it was concluded that "screening had a significant effect on reduction in mortality from carcinoma of the uterus" (13).

WEIGHING THE EVIDENCE

When the evidence regarding cause and effect is conflicting, as is often the case, clinicians must decide where the weight of the evidence lies. Table 11.3 summarizes the different types of evidence for cause, depending on

Table 11.3
Types of Evidence for a Cause-And-Effect Relationship and their Relative Strengths

STRENGTH	DESIGN	FINDING
Strong	Clinical trial	Temporality
↑	Cohort study	Strength
	Case control study	Reversibility
	Cross-sectional	Dose-response
	Aggregate risk[a]	Consistency
	Case series	Biologic
↓	Case report	Plausibility
		Specificity
Weak		Analogy

[a] Aggregate risk studies' strength depends on whether they are multiple time series (strongest), single time series, or cross-sectional (weakest).

research design and the findings of the research itself, and indicates (roughly) relative strengths in helping establish or discard a causal hypothesis.

SUMMARY

Cause-and-effect relationships underlie diagnostic, preventive, and therapeutic activities in clinical medicine.

Diseases usually have many causes, although occasionally one might predominate. Often, several causes interact with one another in such a way that the risk of disease is more than would be expected by simply adding up the effects of the individual causes taken separately.

Causes of disease can be proximal pathogenetic mechanisms or more remote genetic, environmental, or behavioral factors. Medical interventions to prevent or reverse disease can occur at any place in the development of disease, from remote origins to proximal mechanisms.

The case for causation rests primarily on the strength of the research designs used to establish it. Because we rarely have the opportunity to establish cause using randomized controlled trials, observational studies are necessary. In such cases, factors that strengthen the argument for a cause-and-effect relationship include temporal relationships, the strength of the association between cause and effect, the existence of a dose-response relationship, a fall in risk when the purported cause is removed, and consistency of results from several studies. Biologic plausibility and coherence with known facts are other features that help establish cause.

REFERENCES

1. Holmes OW: On the contagiousness of puerperal fever. *N Engl Quart J Med Surg* 1843. In *Medical Classics* 1:207–268, 1936.
2. *Webster's New Collegiate Dictionary*, Springfield, CG Merriam Co, 1977.
3. MacMahon B, Pugh TF. *Epidemiology. Principles and Methods.* Boston, Little, Brown and Co, 1970.
4. Kannel WB. Preventive cardiology. *Postgrad Med* 61:74–85, 1977.
5. Shapiro S, Slone D, Rosenberg L, Kaufman DW, Stolley PD, Miettinen OS: Oral-contraceptive use in relation to myocardial infarction. *Lancet* 1:743–747, 1979.
6. Bradford-Hill AB: The environment and disease: association or causation? *Proc Roy Soc Med* 58:295–300, 1965.
7. *Morbidity and Mortality Weekly Report* 28:1–11, 1979.
8. Beasley RP, Lin CC, Hwang LY, Chien CS: Hepatocellular carcinoma and hepatitis B virus. *Lancet* 2:1129–1133, 1981.
9. Moertel CG, Fleming TR, Rubin J, Kvols LK, Sarna G, Koch R, Currie VE, Young CW, Jones SE, Davignon JP: A clinical trial of amygdalin (laetrile) in the treatment of human cancer. *N Engl J Med* 306:201–206, 1982.
10. St. Leger AS, Cochrane AL, Moore F: Factors associated with cardiac mortality in developed countries with particular reference to the consumption of wine. *Lancet* 1:1017–1020, 1979.
11. Michael M III, Boyce WT, Wilcox AJ: *Biomedical Bestiary: An Epidemiologic Guide to Flaws and Fallacies in the Medical Literature.* Boston, Little, Brown and Co, 1984.
12. *Morbidity and mortality* 30:25–28, 1981.
13. Cervical Cancer Screening Programs: I. Epidemiology and natural history of carcinoma of the cervix. *Can Med Assoc J* 114:1003–1033, 1976.

SUGGESTED READINGS

Bradford-Hill A: The environment and disease: association or causation? *Proc Roy Soc Med* 58:295–300, 1965.

Chalmers AF: *What is this Thing Called Science?* ed 2. New York, University of Queensland Press, 1982.

Evans AS: Causation and disease: a chronological journey. *Am J Epidemiol* 108:249–257, 1978.

Department of Clinical Epidemiology and Biostatistics, McMaster University Health Sciences Centre: How to read clinical journals IV. To determine etiology or causation. *Can Med Assoc J* 124:985–990, 1981.

Weiss NS: Inferring causal relationships: elaboration of the criterion of "dose-response." *Am J Epidemiol* 113:487–490, 1981.

APPENDIX 11.1. MAIN QUESTIONS FOR DETERMINING THE VALIDITY OF STUDIES IN WHICH INCIDENCE RATES ARE COMPARED—TO DESCRIBE RISK FACTORS, CAUSES, PROGNOSTIC FACTORS, AND THE EFFECTS OF THERAPEUTIC OR PREVENTIVE INTERVENTIONS[a]

1. All questions for incidence studies without comparisons
AND
2. *Are compared groups similar.*
   a. At the beginning of follow-up in *susceptibility to the outcome* of interest?
   (Established by one or more of the following: randomization, restriction, matching, stratified analysis, and/or mathematical adjustment)
   b. During follow-up in experiences that might affect outcome except for the factor of interest (*co-interventions*)?
3. *Are outcomes* sought with the same effort, and are their presence established by the same criteria?

---

[a] These questions are not meant to be all-inclusive nor to replace independent, critical thinking. They are rough guidelines, including only the most basic elements of a sound study.

chapter 12

SUMMING UP

Where is the knowledge we have lost in information?

T. S. ELIOT

The validity of clinical research depends on its scientific credibility—its believability to thoughtful, unbiased scientists. Both clinicians, who base their decisions on the medical literature, and researchers, who create it, need to understand what adds to and subtracts from the strength of scientific research.

To judge scientific credibility, readers must take an active role. They must decide what they want to discover in the work and then see if the information is present, accounted for, or neglected. By just reading passively, without considering the basic scientific principles systematically and in advance, one will be less likely to notice shortcomings and more likely to be misled.

This chapter has three parts. First, we will discuss how research articles pertaining to a given clinical question are identified and how their numbers can be reduced to manageable proportions without sacrificing needed information. Next, we will summarize basic rules for judging the strength of individual articles; this section deals with concepts that have been discussed throughout the book. Finally, we will consider how the many articles on a given research question, as a group, are weighted so as to discover where the best available estimate of the truth lies. It is on this estimate that clinicians must base their clinical decisions until better information becomes available.

Whatever the strength of the best available evidence, clinicians must use it both as a basis for action—sometimes rather bold action—at the time, yet regard it as fallible and subject to revision. One scholar has distinguished between "decisions" and "conclusions" (1). We decide something is true if we will act as if it is so, for the present, until better information comes along. Conclusions, on the other hand, are settled issues and are expected to be more durable. Clinicians are mainly concerned with decisions. Moreover, the integrity of the scientific enterprise rests on the willingness of its participants to engage in open-minded, well-informed arguments for and against a current view of the truth, to accept new evidence, and to change their minds.

WHICH ARTICLES ARE IMPORTANT FOR CLINICAL DECISION MAKING?

All articles are not equally important for clinical decision making. Thoughtful clinicians must find and value the soundest articles in the face of an almost overwhelming body of available information.

Figure 12.1 summarizes an approach to distinguishing articles of fundamental importance to clinical decision making from those that are not. Many articles—reviews, teaching articles, editorials—are written to describe what is generally believed to be true, but are not themselves reports of original research aimed at establishing that truth. These articles are a convenient source of summary information, but they are derived from our true knowledge base and are not independent contributions to it. Moreover, they are usually written by people with an established point of view, so that there is the potential for bias.

Other articles describe original research done in laboratories for the purpose of understanding the biology of disease. These studies provide a rich source of hypotheses about health and disease. Yet, "bench" research cannot, in itself, establish with certainty what will happen in humans, because phenomena in actual patients, who are complex organisms in a similarly complex physical and social environment, involve variables that have been deliberately excluded from laboratory experiments.

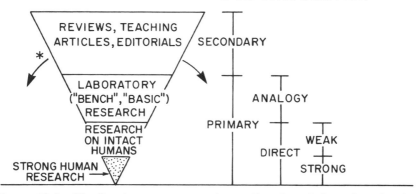

Figure 12.1. The literature on a research question: the relative value of various kinds of articles for answering a clinical question.

Research involving intact humans and intended to guide clinical decision making ("clinical research") is, of course, conducted with varying degrees of scientific rigor. Even by crude standards, most is relatively weak. Few articles involve original research, actual patients, and strong methods.

Throughout this book we have argued that the validity of clinical research depends on the strength of its methods (internal validity) and the extent to which it applies to a particular clinical setting (generalizability). If so, a few good articles are more valuable than many weak or inappropriate ones. Thus, the overall conclusion from the medical literature depends mostly on how a relatively few articles are interpreted. A "review of the literature" should involve selecting these articles carefully, identifying their scientific strengths and weaknesses, and weighing the evidence when, as is often the case, their conclusions differ.

FINDING USEFUL ARTICLES

To review the published literature concerning a clinical question, it is first necessary to sort through a large number of titles, often thousands, in order to find the small number of articles that are useful. The objective is to reduce the literature to manageable proportions without missing important articles. The task can be intimidating and time-consuming. We describe a plan of attack.

The first step is to develop a set of criteria for screening titles so as to select articles that may be relevant while excluding a much larger number that clearly are not. The criteria should define a sensitive test for the articles that one hopes to find in the same sense as a screening test should be sensitive for a disease—that is, few useful articles should be missed. If necessary, specificity can be sacrificed to achieve sensitivity, with the understanding that it will be necessary to evaluate many "false positive" articles in more detail for each one that meets the final criteria. Often a useful screening algorithm is defined by the joint occurrence of a few key words in the title—for example, sarcoidosis/pulmonary/corticosteroid or cancer/pancreatic/diagnosis (or ultrasound). Usually, more than one set of screening criteria and more than one source of titles—for example, key words and the citation index for classic references—are used.

Second, the screening criteria are applied to lists of journal titles. If there is time, it is best to consult several lists, with complementary strengths and weaknesses. One can examine large data bases—Index Medicus and others—in bound volumes or search them by computer in most medical libraries. Literature searches can also be accomplished on home computers, for those willing to invest the time and the money to learn and obtain software and service. Other sources of titles are recent review articles, other articles on the same topic, textbooks, and suggestions from experts in the field.

The result of this search is a large number of titles, some of which represent relevant articles and many of which do not.

Third, one must apply specific criteria in order to identify the articles that are actually appropriate for the question at hand. Three kinds of criteria are often used:

- Does the article address the specific clinical question that was the reason for the search in the first place?
- Does the article represent original research, not secondary information or opinion?
- Is the research based on relatively strong methods? For example, for questions of cause, one might exclude case reports.

Many inappropriate articles can be ruled out in a series of simple steps. For articles that have been identified by an algorithm during a computerized search, some can be excluded by examination of the full title. For example, in a search for articles about the elderly, the presence of the synonym "older" could cause an article suggesting that a pediatric disease occurs more often in older children to appear. Other titles can be excluded because they are in journals that do not publish original research. Sometimes abstracts are included in data bases and contain enough information to exclude an article.

Fourth, one must actually look at the text of the articles that remain to see which meet the final criteria. By this time, the number of articles has been reduced enough that the task is feasible.

If there is not sufficient time for a full, broadly based search for articles, the first step of this process can be abbreviated. One can examine only those lists of titles that are most accessible and are expected to have the highest yield, such as recent review or research articles and textbooks (remembering that textbooks were sent to press several months before publication and become increasingly out-of-date after that time). By restricting the breadth of this search, we may miss some important articles, but the increased feasibility may be worth the risk.

Figure 12.2 summarizes these steps and illustrates the search process for a specific question: the causes of iatrogenic illness in the elderly (2).

JUDGING INDIVIDUAL ARTICLES

Raising and Testing Hypotheses

The conclusions of an individual piece of research fall on a spectrum of believability according to the decisiveness of the scientific strategy used. At one end of the spectrum are reports that only suggest relationships, albeit potentially useful ones, about health and disease, without putting these ideas to the test. Most case reports serve this function. The conclusions of these studies are tentative; many are later refuted. At the other end of the spectrum are studies—for example, large randomized controlled trials—that have put ideas to a rigorous test. Conclusions from these studies are more definitive. Most studies fall between these extremes.

A priori hypotheses are important. Without them, false positive findings can make their way into the literature in the following way. Suppose one

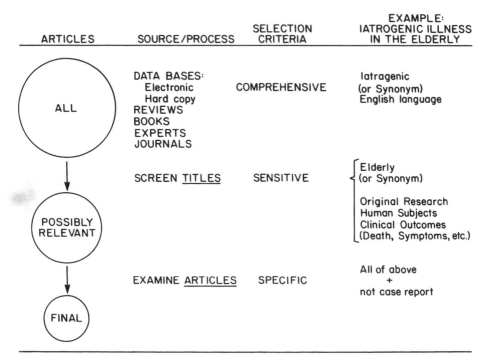

Figure 12.2. Literature search: identifying the few most important articles from the medical literature as a whole. (Example from Fletcher RH, Fletcher SW: *Iatrogenic illness and the Elderly*, in press.)

examines a data set in which none of the variables is associated with any of the others in nature—that is, in the population from which came the particular sample being studied. As discussed in Chapter 9, if a large number of comparisons are made, measures of association—for example, relative risk—for some of them will be extreme enough to appear "real," even though the associations are only by chance. At a conventional level of statistical significance, $p < .05$, 1 in 20 such comparisons will be statistically significant, by definition. Of course, the observed associations are real for the particular data set at hand—but not necessarily in the population—because the current sample may misrepresent all such samples from the population of interest.

Now suppose that one of these comparisons is selected out of the larger set of all possible comparisons and given special emphasis, perhaps because it fits well with existing theories or is otherwise particularly interesting. Suppose the other comparisons are not mentioned in the final report. Then the association, taken out of context, can appear very real. This process— random (chance) occurrence of associations followed by biased selection of interesting ones—is not unusual in published research.

There are several clues that signal the degree to which a given study is *hypothesis testing*, rather than *hypothesis raising* (Table 12.1).

The first, a strong research design, is not a strictly separate factor from the others. Making hypotheses in advance and limiting the number of comparisons examined are aimed at reducing the number of apparently "significant" comparisons that emerge from a study. The investigator can "call the shots" beforehand by naming which of many research questions are of primary importance and what their answers should be—that is, they can make hypotheses. If the *a priori* hypotheses are confirmed, one can place more confidence in the findings. Alternatively, investigators can simply limit the number of comparisons made after the fact, so that there is less chance of false positive findings for the study as a whole. Or they can insist on a particularly small p value for individual findings, on the understanding that the reported p values for each are an underestimate of the role of chance in these findings.

Another strategy is to raise hypotheses on one set of data and test them on a separate one (Figure 12.3). This process is illustrated in the following example.

Example—Fischl et al. developed an index, including seven physical signs, for predicting the early recurrence of acute asthma after discharge from an emergency

Table 12.1
Characteristics of a Study that Determine whether it can Test or only Raise Hypotheses

CHARACTERISTIC	HYPOTHESIS RAISING	HYPOTHESIS TESTING
Design	Weak	Strong
Hypotheses	None (or after data collected and analysed)	Stated before study begun
Comparisons	Many	Few
P-value	Large	Small
Results confirmed on separate data set	No	Yes

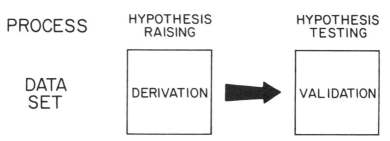

Figure 12.3. Developing a hypothesis on one data set and testing it on another.

department (3). Among 205 patients at the investigators' medical center, patients from whom the index was developed, the index had a sensitivity of 95% and a specificity of 97%. The results were so striking that the index began to be put into clinical practice elsewhere.

Later, two groups of investigators independently tested the index in other settings (4, 5). The results were disappointing. The sensitivity and specificity were 40% and 71%, respectively, in one study and 18.1% and 82.4% in the other.

These studies illustrate the dangers of placing too much confidence in a relationship that has been suggested in one data set but not tested in another, independent one. There are several possible reasons for the difference in performance. Patients in the original sample might have misrepresented all patients in that setting through either biased selection or chance, patients in other settings might be systematically different, or the index might have been applied differently, despite efforts to use it in the same way.

Whatever the strategies used to increase the hypothesis-testing character of a study, it is the author's responsibility to make it clear where a particular study stands on the hypotheses-raising/hypothesis-testing spectrum and why. The readers' task is to seek out this information or reconstruct it, if it is not apparent. However, one should not eschew studies that mainly raise hypotheses.

Design of Individual Studies

This book has described the scientific principles by which clinical research is judged. It is not possible to summarize all of the factors that affect the validity of research. However, some features are so fundamental that they are almost necessary, though not sufficient, standards for validity.

We have outlined basic criteria for the scientific credibility of specific research designs in the Appendices to several chapters. At the end of Chapter 1, we summarize a set of questions that should be asked of most studies—by investigators and readers alike. They concern the nature of the research question, the generalizability and clinical usefulness of the results, and two processes that can affect internal validity: bias and chance. In later chapters, we consider groundrules for studies of diagnosis, prevalence, incidence, treatment, and cause.

Taken together, these appendices describe basic issues that should be considered when deciding whether an article might be sufficiently strong to be useful in a literature review (above) and in setting criteria to assign weights to articles when preparing a synthesis of the results of several articles (below).

Does the Design Fit the Question?

One cannot speak of "good" or "bad" research designs in general without reference to the question they are intended to answer. Table 12.2 matches clinical questions to the best research designs used to answer them. The

Table 12.2
Matching the Strongest Research Designs to Clinical Questions

QUESTION	DESIGN
Diagnosis	Prevalence
Prevalence	Prevalence
Incidence	Cohort
Risk	Cohort
	Case control
Prognosis	Cohort
Treatment	Clinical trial
Cause	Cohort
	Case control

table is meant to offer guidelines; it should not preclude creative but scientifically sound approaches other than those listed.

SUMMARIZING THE RESULTS OF MANY STUDIES

The current state of knowledge on a question is usually decided by the pattern of results from all studies addressing the question, rather than by one definitive study. The commonest way of establishing this pattern is by implicit judgment—that is, opinion, without having stated in advance the groundrules by which the contributions of individual studies would be weighted. Judgments of this sort often take the form of a traditional ("narrative") review article by an expert in the relevant field or a consensus of scholars representing the many points of view that bear on a question— for example, the National Institutes of Health's Consensus Development Conferences.

In recent years, a variety of more structured methods of summarizing published research have been developed and have gained popularity. These methods have the advantage of making explicit the assumptions behind the weight assigned to the various studies. They also follow the scientific method more directly: setting criteria in advance, gathering data (in this case, the results of individual studies), and allowing the conclusions to follow from the criteria and data.

The process of summing up the research on a question, using structured methods, is referred to as *meta-analysis*—literally, analysis of analysis—or *information synthesis*. This approach is particularly useful when there is one specific question and at least a few relatively strong studies that come to different conclusions. The method has so far been applied mainly to clinical trials.

There are two general approaches to meta-analysis. One is to weigh the importance attached to individual studies according to how well they meet predetermined methodological criteria. The other is to summarize, quantitatively, the results of many studies to form, in effect, one large study with more statistical power than any of the individual studies alone.

Criteria-Based Analysis of the Literature

Published articles on a question can be summarized by judging the methods of individual studies against basic standards for scientific credibility. Appendices at the end of several chapters are examples of these criteria for the several kinds of clinical questions discussed in this book.

The basic steps in a criteria-based meta-analysis are:

1. Select a single clinical question.
2. Identify the published studies bearing on this question.
3. Set criteria for scientific credibility according to the nature of the question. For example, to determine the efficiency of a drug one should have a treated and comparison group, equal susceptibility to the outcomes of interest (other than the effects of treatment), unbiased assessment of outcomes, etc.
4. Determine how individual studies meet the methodological standard.
5. See if there is a relationship between the scientific credibility of the studies and their conclusions.

Often, there is a relationship between the extent to which individual studies meet basic criteria for sound methods and the conclusions of these studies.

Example—Although Bacille Calmette-Guerin (BCG) vaccine has been used to prevent tuberculosis for over 50 years and is required in many countries, its efficacy is controversial. In part this is because the several large-scale clinical trials to evaluate BCG have reported conflicting results. Clemens et al. compared the methods used in these trials to their results (6). Their findings are summarized in Table 12.3 and Figure 12.4. The investigators interpret their results as showing that "adequate demonstration of unbiased detection of tuberculosis was available only for the three trials reporting 75% or greater efficacy; and ... in most trials reporting low efficacy, the results had wide confidence intervals that could not exclude high efficacy, but the trials reporting high efficacy all had narrow confidence intervals that excluded low efficacy." The authors concluded that BCG can confer protection and that "bias or inadequate statistical power may have contributed to the conflicting data."

Criteria-based analyses of the literature are relatively crude. Failures to meet criteria are often counted as either present or absent, and a study's overall soundness may be summarized by the proportion of criteria met. Some criteria might be more important to the study's validity than others; failure to meet some individual criteria may be sufficient to disqualify the results altogether. So the results of this form of meta-analysis can only be taken as a guide—albeit a compelling guide if one accepts the criteria for methodological soundness and that methodological soundness determines the validity of results.

Table 12.3
Protection Against Bias and Adequacy of Statistical Precision in Eight Major BCG Trials[a]

| TRIAL | ADEQUATE PROTECTION AGAINST | | | | ADEQUATE STATISTICAL PRECISION? | OBSERVED PROTECTIVE EFFICACY |
	SUSCEPTI-BILITY BIAS?	SURVEIL-LANCE BIAS?	DIAG-NOSTIC TESTING BIAS?	DIAGNOS-TIC IN-TERPRETA-TION BIAS?		
						%
North American Indians	Yes	Yes	Yes	Yes	Yes	80
England	Yes	Yes	Yes	Yes	Yes	76
Chicago	Probable	Yes	Yes	Yes	Yes	75
Puerto Rico	Yes	No	No	No	No	29
Madanapalle	Equivocal	No	No	Probable	No	20
Georgia-Alabama	Yes	No	No	Equivocal	No	6
Chingleput	Probable	No	No	Yes	Yes	-32
Georgia	Yes	No	No	No	No	-56

[a] See text for explanation.

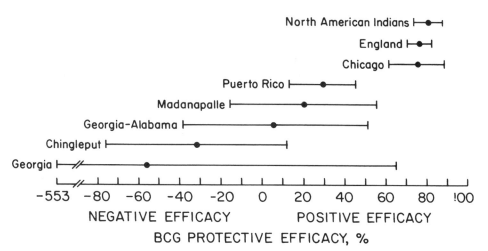

Figure 12.4. Protection against bias and adequacy of statistical power in eight major BCG trials. (From Clemens JD, Chuong JH, Feinstein AR: The BCG controversy. A methodological and statistical reappraisal. 249:2362–2369, 1983.)

Pooling

Not uncommonly, the results of various individual studies are indecisive because each study describes too few patients or too few outcome events. Consequently, estimates of rates from these studies are unstable, and comparisons of rates run an unacceptably high risk of missing true effects (Type II error).

Pooling refers to the process of aggregating the results of several relatively small studies of the same question to form, in effect, one large one. Sometimes, the contributions of individual studies to the overall result are weighted according to their size.

The advantage of pooling is that it can result in adequate statistical power to detect meaningful differences if they exist. Pooling is particularly useful when the disease and/or the outcome events of interest occur infrequently. Under these circumstances there are no other feasible ways to achieve statistical power.

Example—There are many reports of peptic ulcer disease during corticosteroid therapy. Yet, it has been difficult to establish, by means of observational studies, whether corticosteroids cause ulcers because many of the situations in which they are given—for example, during stress and in conjunction with gastric-irritating drugs—may themselves predispose to peptic ulcer disease. Also, ulcers may be sought more diligently in patients receiving corticosteroids and go undetected in other patients.

Randomized controlled trials are the best way to determine cause and effect. Although it is not possible to allocate randomly an intervention that is only harmful, there have been many randomized trials in which corticosteroids were used to treat various conditions and peptic ulcer disease was a side effect. None of these studies was large enough in itself to test the corticosteroid/ulcer hypothesis.

In one review of 71 controlled trials of corticosteroids in which patients were randomized (or its equivalent) and peptic ulcer disease was considered, there were about 86 patients and one case of peptic ulcer disease per study; only 31 of the trials reported any patients with ulcers. The investigators pooled the results of these 71 trials to obtain sufficient statistical power. In the pooled study, there were 6111 patients and about 80 ulcers. The rate of peptic ulcer disease was 1.8 in the corticosteroid group and 0.8 in the control group (relative risk 2.3, 95% confidence interval 1.4–3.7).

The pooled results might have been misleading because individual studies used different definitions of eligible patients, exposure to corticosteroids, and peptic ulcer disease. However, the results were similar when examined separately according to the presence and absence of other risk factors and by various doses, routes of administration, duration of therapy, and whether the disease was suspected, defined as bleeding, or specifically diagnosed.

Thus, the combined results of many studies, each with relatively sound design but too small to answer the question, gave sufficient statistical power to detect risk. Pooling provided evidence that corticosteroid therapy causes peptic ulcer disease— although infrequently (7).

Opponents of pooling argue that the ways in which patients, interventions, and outcomes were selected in the various studies are so dissimilar that it is not reasonable to combine them. "Splitters" are not as satisfied with pooling as "lumpers."

Also, pooling deals only with statistical power. It does not correct for whatever biases existed in the designs of the various individual studies, nor can it be assumed that these biases cancel each other out when the studies are aggregated.

PUBLICATION AND BIAS

As does everyone else, physicians prefer good news. Thus, such words as "efficacy," "predicting," and "correlation" are the order of the day in journal titles. It is considerably less appealing to contemplate things that do not work. In fact, such observations are often considered failures. Researchers with the bad fortune to make such observations are likely to be advised by their friends, with gentle malice, to seek publication in the "Journal of Negative Results."

It may be that our penchant for positive results leads to bias in the kinds of articles selected for publication in medical journals. Consider a population of all potential articles—the result of all research carried to completion. Of these, some will find no effect. These negative studies might be less likely to be submitted for publication because their results are often regarded as less interesting. Of the articles submitted for publication, a larger proportion of those with negative results might be rejected by the editorial process for the same reason. The outcome of this process would be that articles actually reaching publication are a biased sample of all research findings, tending to represent efforts to find causes, diagnostic tests, and treatments as being more effective than they actually are.

There are few studies of publication bias. But few who are involved in selecting manuscripts for publication, including authors, reviewers, and editors, doubt its existence. Certainly there is no reason to assert that biased judgments are made deliberately. Everyone does his or her part to put the "best" work forward, but publication is not a random process. There are forces favoring positive over negative results that are quite independent of the relative proportions of these results among all research projects undertaken. Readers should be aware of this bias, lest they become unrealistically impressed with the many new and promising findings that appear in medical journals.

One way to avoid this bias is to give more credibility to large studies than to small ones because most large studies, having required great effort and expense in their execution, will be published regardless of whether they have a positive or negative finding. Smaller studies, requiring less investment, are more easily discarded in the selection process.

DIFFERENT ANSWERS: THE SAME QUESTIONS?

Until now, we have emphasized how studies can come to different conclusions because they have different methods, better for some than for others. But there is an alternative explanation: The research questions, although superficially the same, may actually be fundamentally different. Rather than one or the other study being misleading, both might be right. It may be that human biology, not research methods, accounts for the difference.

Example—Postmenopausal estrogens have long been suspected of causing cardiovascular disease, in part because oral contraceptives are known to be a risk factor in premenopausal women. In 1985, two articles about the cardiovascular risks of postmenopausal estrogens appeared together in the *New England Journal of Medicine.* Both were large cohort studies, involving relatively sound measures of exposure and disease, over 90% follow-up, and adjustment of results for known risk factors for cardiovascular disease, including age, cigarette smoking, hypertension, and serum lipid levels.

One study concluded that estrogens *increased* the risk of cardiovascular disease in postmenopausal women; the adjusted relative risk was 1.76 for total cardiovascular disease and 2.27 for cerebrovascular disease (both $p < .01$) (8). The other study concluded that postmenopausal estrogens *protect* against cardiovascular disease (9). This latter study reported an adjusted relative risk of coronary disease of 0.5 (0.3, 0.8) for women who had ever used postmenopausal estrogens and 0.3 (0.2, 0.6) for women who were currently using the drug.

How can this contradiction be resolved? Although the methods were not beyond reproach, it is difficult to understand how bias might explain such different conclusions. But the exposure to estrogens was quite different in the two studies. One defined exposure as taking estrogens during the 8 years *before* follow-up began; many women were no longer taking estrogens during the period of observation. The other study assessed the effects of exposure *during* follow-up. It has been suggested that the two studies' findings are not inconsistent if estrogens protect against cardiovascular disease while they are taken, and there is an excess in rates after they are stopped.

Although the relationship between postmenopausal estrogens and cardiovascular disease is not yet understood, these studies, because of their relatively strong methods and their overtly different findings, illustrate the possibility that biologic factors may explain the contradiction.

Studies of cause and effect that seem to be asking similar questions can in fact present different questions in at least four ways: The patients, interventions, follow-up, and end results may not be the same. Differences among studies in any one of these may be enough to give different results.

READING JOURNALS

So far in this chapter, we have discussed how one might undertake an indepth review of an individual article or a set of articles bearing on a clinical question. Yet, most of us also approach the literature in another way. We subscribe to journals and try to "read" them, as best we can, in limited periods of time. Or we gather many articles on a specific clinical question and review them. Both involve dealing with a large number of articles in a short time.

Can clinical epidemiology help us do this? We believe it can. As we pointed out earlier, many articles are not worth much time from the general reader either because they are not relevant to the clinician's work or are not done well enough. Using the principles of clinical epidemiology, one can eliminate these articles, usually in the moments it takes to scan a 150-word abstract.

Many danger signals of a poor study are easily recognized. For example,

- A negative clinical trial based on a small number of patients (strong possibility of a false negative result);
- An evaluation of a diagnostic test in which patients with negative test results are not evaluated further (no information or false negative test results);
- A description of the natural history of disease based on the experience of patients currently attending a teaching hospital clinic (a "survival cohort" and also a biased sample of all patients with the condition).

Signals of a potentially good study can also be easy to recognize, for example:

- Any large randomized controlled trial;
- Studies of a diagnostic test in which the true presence or absence of disease is carefully established.

Journal readers should take an active role in judging each article. First, they should decide what they expect from the article, given the question it addresses. Then they see if the article provides it. It is much less effective to read the article and then ask if it was satisfactory. It is too easy to become beguiled by what is said, forgetting what should have been said.

We recommend the sets of questions summarized in the appendices to the chapters in this book. Asking them will help you identify the few articles that are worth more time.

With this approach or a comparable one, clinicians can gain both efficiency and knowledge. Moreover, they can have the satisfaction of knowing that they are prepared for the work and to do it well.

REFERENCES

1. Tukey JW: Conclusions and decisions. *Technometrics* 2:423–433, 1960.
2. Fletcher RH, Fletcher SW. *Iatrogenic Illness and the Elderly.* (in press).
3. Fischl MA, Pitchenik A, Gardner LB: An index predicting relapse and need for hospitalization in patients with acute bronchial asthma. *N Engl J Med* 305:783–789, 1981.
4. Rose CC, Murphy JG, Schwartz JS: Performance of an index predicting the response of patients with acute bronchial asthma to intensive emergency department treatment. *N Engl J Med* 310:573–577, 1984.
5. Centor RM, Yarbrough B, Wood JP: Inability to predict relapse in acute asthma. *N Engl J Med* 310:577–580, 1984.
6. Clemens JD, Chuong JH, Feinstein AR: The BCG controversy. A methodological and statistical reappraisal. *JAMA* 249:2362–2369, 1983.

7. Messer J, Reitman D, Sacks HS, Smith H Jr, Chalmers TC: Association of adrenocorticosteroid therapy and peptic-ulcer disease. *N Engl J Med* 309:21–24, 1983.
8. Wilson PWF, Garrison RJ, Castelli WP: Postmenopausal estrogen use, cigarette smoking, and cardiovascular morbidity in women over 50. The Framingham Study. *N Engl J Med* 313:1038–1043, 1985.
9. Stampfer MJ, Willett WC, Colditz GA, Rosner B, Speizer FE, Hennekens CH: A prospective study of postmenopausal estrogen therapy and coronary heart disease. *N Engl J Med* 313:1044–1049, 1985.

SUGGESTED READINGS

Elashoff JD: Combining the results of clinical trials (Editorial). *Gastroenterology* 75:1170–1172, 1978.

Epidemiology Work Group of the Interagency Regulatory Liason Group: Guidelines for documentation of epidemiologic studies. *Am J Epidemiol* 114:609–713, 1981.

Goldschmidt PG: Information synthesis: a practical guide. *Health Services Res* 21:215–237, 1986.

Haynes RB, McKibbon KA, Walker CJ, Mousseau J, Baker LM, Fitzgerald D, Guyatt G, Norman GR: Computer searching of the medical literature: an evaluation of MEDLINE searching systems. *Ann Intern Med* 103:812–816, 1985.

Haynes RB, McKibbon KA, Fitzgerald D, Guyatt GH, Walker CJ, Sackett DL: How to keep up with the medical literature: 1. Why try to keep up and how to get started. *Ann Intern Med* 105:149–153, 1986.

Haynes RB, McKibbon KA, Fitzgerald D, Guyatt GH, Walker CJ, Sackett DL: How to keep up with the medical literature: II. Deciding which journals to read regularly. *Ann Intern Med* 105:309–312, 1986.

Haynes RB, McKibbon KA, Fitzgerald D, Guyatt GH, Walker CJ, Sackett DL: How to keep up with the medical literature: III. Expanding the number of journals you read regularly. *Ann Intern Med* 105:474–478, 1986.

Haynes RB, McKibbon KA, Fitzgerald D, Guyatt GH, Walker CJ, Sackett DL: How to keep up with the medical literature: IV. Using the literature to solve clinical problems. *Ann Intern Med* 105:636–640, 1986.

Light RJ, Pillemer DB: *Summing Up. The Science of Reviewing Research.* Cambridge, MA, Harvard University Press, 1984.

Petersdorf RG: The pathogenesis of fraud in medical science. *Ann Intern Med* 104:252–254, 1986.

Wolf FM: Meta-analysis. Quantitative methods for research synthesis. Series No. 07-059. Beverly Hills, Sage, 1986.

INDEX